PRACTICE MADE PERFECT

PRACTICE MADE PERFECT

THE PHYSICIAN'S GUIDE TO COMMUNICATION AND MARKETING

Edna Kaplan

Barrington Press / Boston / Massachusetts

Printed in the United States of America

Published by Barrington Press
P. O. Box 291
Boston University Station
Boston, Massachusetts 02215

10 9 8 7 6 5 4 3 2 1

Library of Congress Cataloging in Publication Data

Kaplan, Edna, date.
Practice made perfect.

Includes bibliographical references.
Includes index.
1. Physician and patient. 2. Interpersonal communication.
3. Medicine—Practice. 4. Medical care—Marketing. I. Title.
R727.3.K33 1990
610.69'6—dc20 89-18198
ISBN 0-9616920-1-4

The author is grateful to publishers and authors for permission to reprint material from the following:

Advertising Research Foundation for "Consumers' Attitudes Toward Accountants, Lawyers and Physicians with Respect to Advertising Professional Services" by R. Hite and J. Bellizi, *Journal of Advertising Research* Vol. 26 p. 45, © 1986.

Acknowledgments of permissions continue following the index.

ACKNOWLEDGMENTS

Nearly everyone I have ever worked with has in some way helped me write this book, but there are a few people to whom I owe special debts of gratitude. Most of all, I am grateful to my husband Don, who not only inspires me, but also took the children skiing almost every weekend to allow me writing time. I am grateful too to my sons, Jonathan and Scott, for their good humored self-sufficiency, and to all my family and friends for their unwavering support. I would like to express my deep appreciation to Dr. Otto Lerbinger for his continued encouragement and insightful direction during the writing of this book. Last, but not least, I am grateful to Beth Lerbinger and Ginny O'Brien, whose patience and judicious editing made this book better than it might have been.

CONTENTS

INTRODUCTION

> With public sentiment, nothing can fail;
> without it, nothing can succeed
> *Abraham Lincoln*

Practice Made Perfect: The Physician's Guide to Communication and Marketing provides today's physician with the means to bring into public view the humaneness inherent in the choice of medicine as a career. By more effective use of communication tools, the climate for medical practice—in one's office, community, and country—can be improved, to the mutual benefit of physicians and patients. This book presents effective strategies for all physicians, not only for those who wish to expand their practices.

Based on over two hundred interviews and written reports by physicians and many of the leading experts in the fields of public relations, practice management, and marketing, this book offers concise, detailed, practical advice on how to use various communication vehicles to make the private practice of medicine a rewarding career. It covers a broad range of subjects, including how to use communication strategies to attract patients and keep them satisfied, how to stay ahead of the competition (when and if the need arises), how to make accurate diagnoses more quickly, and how to shape medical careers to make the work more enjoyable. The role physicians can play in shaping public attitudes toward health care delivery is also discussed, as are getting media attention and responding appropriately to it.

The communication techniques used by fee-for-service medical practices today range from conservative to aggressive. This book is arranged accordingly, with communication tools examined and evaluated from the standpoint of attaining each physician's professional and personal goals, while at the same time maintaining medicine's reputation and the profession's traditional service orientation.

Practice Made Perfect: The Physician's Guide to Communication and Marketing is also for practice management, public relations, and marketing consultants who are seeking physicians as clients. The needs of fee-for-service physicians differ from those of hospitals, health maintenance organizations, and medical associations. In many respects, serving the needs of medical practices is a new frontier, one that is likely to expand rapidly in coming years. My analysis of current health care public relations, marketing and advertising practices aims at providing insight into a growing trend—the marketing of medical professionals.

Part I

THE NEW REALITY

1 THE NEW REALITY
2 WHY COMMUNICATE?

1 THE NEW REALITY

In the fall of 1987, a "Today Show" segment featured the man voted 1987 Doctor of the Year by the American Academy of Family Physicians. Dr. Leeon F. Aller of Washington State was an impressive recipient. Not only did he have a thriving practice in family medicine, but he was also a teacher of medicine and a humanitarian in the Albert Schweitzer tradition. Each year he volunteered his services at a clinic in Guatemala. He and his wife had adopted several children and taken in numerous foster children. Dr. Aller had been a scoutmaster and founded a prison ministry in an attempt to "bring out the good things in people."

It was an upbeat report, portraying the doctor as a selfless, kind human being who was appreciated and adored by his patients. But the commentator's remarks were jarring. "Whenever I do a report like this," he said, "I am invariably asked, 'Why can't my doctor be like that?'" The commentator's advice to viewers: "If you don't like your doctor, find another one. There are thousands of family doctors out there." The message was clear. "Good" doctors have to be sought out, shopped for. They may not be easy to find.

The commentator's remarks, though discordant, reflect the widely held view that the physician dedicated to service is becoming increasingly rare. And many Americans, no longer content to settle for a physician perceived to be uncaring, are switching providers with little hesitation. Health care, once a seller's market, is rapidly becoming a buyer's market.

Medicine is changing, as is the climate for medical practice, and the environment for practicing medicine is no longer as hospitable as it once was. For American physicians, the stakes are high. How medicine is practiced in the 1990s and beyond is largely dependent on public opinion. Will the private practice of medicine go the way of the corner grocery store, fading in the face of costs and competition, or will public opinion favor its continuation?

Doctors readily admit that there is a need to re-establish confidence in and understanding of their profession. They recognize that their job begins with doctor-patient relationships and that it is measured by the degree of public confidence reflected in the doctor image.

The Impact of Economics

The perception that caring physicians are a dying breed stems in large part from the dramatic changes that have swept the medical profession in the past forty years. A rapid growth in scale and scope has brought changes that have revolutionized the private practice of medicine, according to Arnold Relman, editor of the *New England Journal of Medicine.* Once a cottage industry characterized by trusting doctor-patient relationships, medicine has become a vast enterprise increasingly driven by economic considerations. In 1980 health care in the United States accounted for 9.1 percent of the gross national product. By the year 2000, health care expenditures may reach 14 percent of GNP, the Health Care Financing Administration forecasts.

With the United Kingdom and Japan enjoying comparable health status for 5.5 percent of GNP, and Canada, a society much like our own, holding it at 7 percent of GNP, it is no wonder that the value and role of medicine in our society have been undergoing a reappraisal.

Changes in the way physicians are reimbursed are among the factors that have led to closer public scrutiny of health care financing. Much of physicians' income now comes from Medicare and Medicaid, programs funded by tax dollars. In 1975 physicians' fees accounted for 5 percent of health care expenditures; in 1988 they accounted for 20 percent of total medical costs. And whereas the government financed 26 percent of health care expenditures in 1968, by 1988 it was financing 41 percent. The combined cost of Medicare and Medicaid programs doubled every four years between 1965 and 1985, according to the Center for Economic Development.

Because these programs are publicly financed, they have caught the interest of journalists, politicians, and the public. That interest has brought with it public examination of medical practice, and the appraisal has not always been favorable. Often, the presumption is that doctors' fees are the major factor in driving up costs.

As a result, America's physicians find themselves under attack, their dedication to service questioned. A review of data from several surveys suggests that while the public's satisfaction with the quality of health care has not yet been affected by changes in the health care system, citizens appear to be both more litigious and more critical and scrutinizing of doctors' behavior than they were in the past.

A Drop in Esteem

According to a Gallup poll, Americans in the early 1980s gave doctors high ratings for contributing to the general good of society, placing them second only to the clergy. Doctors were deemed to have more prestige and status than other professionals in their communities—59 percent of the public gave them top ratings. Compared to twenty-three other occupational groups, physicians ranked second, after the clergy, for their honesty and ethical standards.

By the mid-1980s, however, things had changed. Opinion surveys indicated that the public was angry with physicians and did not hold the profession in as high esteem as it had in the past. American Medical Association polls in the late 1980s indicated that the public harbored considerable negative sentiment toward physicians. Fully 64 percent of those polled said people were beginning to lose faith in doctors, a number that has remained stable but uncomfortably high. Another 49 percent agreed with the statement "Doctors don't care about people as much as they used to." In a discussion of these findings, a Sunday *New York Times Magazine* article by Daniel Okrent referred to the "unhappy human relationships with physicians."

Tomorrow's Doctors

The medical establishment has recognized this new reality. Medical education must change, medical educators state, for the doctors of tomorrow to be perceived as more caring and humane. The educators are urging doctors to show more visible concern for society and to voice their social conscience. They are calling for reforms in medical training that put greater emphasis on community service and doctor-patient relationship skills.

In a show of near unanimity, according to Dr. David Rogers of the New York Academy of Medicine, thirty-one of the country's leading medical educators, participating in a national seminar on medical education, agreed that:

- Our nation needs doctors with a broader and more sensitive view of the role and place of medicine in society.
- Doctors must become more skillful in doctor-patient relationships.
- Doctors should pay more attention to health promotion, disease prevention, and the social, environmental, and emotional factors bearing on health.
- Doctors should have a strong sense of social responsibility for the health and medical care rendered in their communities.

For these recommendations to be implemented, future medical school curricula will have to include courses in communication that will teach tomorrow's doctors the skills needed for effective and satisfying doctor-patient relationships and for promoting health in their communities.

Medical educators are already experimenting within the medical system. Harvard University's School of Medicine introduced a revamped curriculum in the 1987-1988 academic year. Under the new system, some members of the entering class begin clinical rotations in their first year. The goal of the increased clinical exposure is to equip future physicians with better interpersonal skills, which educators now say are as important as scientific knowledge and which also require practice. In New York State, educators have recommended sweeping changes in medical education that would dramatically reduce training in specialties in favor of emphasis on primary care.

"We really do believe the great physicians are excellent scientists, excellent at the biotechnical capacity of medicine, and excellent at healing—at the humanistic side of medicine," said Harvard's Dr. Gordon Moore in discussing the rationale for the new curriculum during a December 1988 *NOVA* broadcast.

"I think we're trying to come back to the old days in a certain way. After all, the doctor was viewed kind of the same way as the teacher, the rabbi, or the priest. He or she was a confidant, a person you could talk to and would get wise counsel from and would understand what you're all about, that you were more than a mass of organs, and would be someone to whom you could turn when there was trouble . . . . That's a wonderful model . . . . We're trying to bring that back, I think, in part," Dr. Thomas Delbanco, director of general medicine at Boston's Beth Israel Hospital, said on the same *NOVA* program.

These changes will presumably improve the climate for medical practice in the future. But what of today's doctors?

Adapting to a More Hostile Environment

Doctors say that recent years have seen the demise of the art of medicine. They point to the public's expectations of wrongdoing by physicians, the growing number of malpractice suits, and the "sins" of some doctors, for example, pride and greed, that erode the doctor image. They point to the need for their ranks to be more enterprising in shaping the evolving health care delivery system. "It is critical that physicians take a proactive role in the design and development of health care delivery systems that will allow the preservation of the physician-patient relationship and the delivery of quality health care," Dr. Joseph Stankaitis of the State University of New York wrote following his study of current issues facing the medical profession.[1] "It is," he said, "a matter of survival."

Physicians sense that the road ahead is a difficult one. Despite economic gains in recent years, physicians, health care analysts, and government officials, citing a physician glut and a trend toward further cost containment, anticipate that physician incomes will decline. A *Medical Economics* poll found doctors to be skeptical about their economic future. Of physicians in solo and group practice, one in three expected earnings to drop. Of eighteen medical specialties represented in the survey, doctors in twelve of these expected earnings to fall off.[2]

Physicians in private practice, however, are far less concerned with income than with loss of autonomy and the potential decline in quality of care. Much of their pessimism is also due to increasingly stifling government regulation, a more litigious society, and growing competition from corporate health care entities.

Need for Action

Their wariness of the future is making physicians realize the need for action on two fronts: public opinion and their own practices. Specialization, technological advances, and alternative health care delivery systems have all had profound effects on the way they practice medicine. Largely through the efforts of their medical associations, physicians are attempting to convince the public that they continue to maintain a service orientation geared toward providing the best available health care at a reasonable cost.

However, with their income threatened, competition increasing, and their image tarnished, there is also a sense among doctors of wanting to do something about their practices, according to Susan Tellem, president of a California public relations firm that specializes in medical practices. Caught between their historic role as service providers and the new reality of a more competitive environment, between the need to stay atop rapid developments in medical treatment and patient demands on their time, physicians have had to give at least some consideration to medical practice as a business. Like other service providers, doctors are struggling to adapt to a new environment in which patients' wants as well as their medical needs must be considered.

With its twenty-four-century history of altruism, the medical profession has generally avoided the business arena, with its focus on bottom-line economics. Medicine, particularly as organized into solo and group practice, has been slow to consider itself a business, and management of the practice has put greater emphasis on the scheduling of patients than on establishing competitive advantage.

Traditionally, there has been little utilization of and a great deal of confusion about the efficacy of the marketing and communication tools used by profit-oriented businesses for enhancing medical practices.

But in growing numbers, physicians are hiring marketing, public relations, and advertising experts to maintain or improve their patient base, to better communicate with patients, to promote new and floundering practices, to help find market niches, and to reshape unrewarding careers.

Some consultants, who say that medicine is a business like any other, are telling doctors to heed the "bias for action" and "stay close to the customer" advice given to other businesses in Thomas Peters and Robert Waterman's best-seller, *In Search of Excellence*. Yet the business and promotional tools that work well for some portions of the service sector may erode rather than enhance the medical practice. Because medicine differs significantly from other, profit-driven businesses in the service sector, and even from other professional services such as law and accounting, solutions to such problems as attracting and keeping patients are not as evident as those for the more bottom-line-oriented service providers.

One principle that does, indeed, apply equally to business and medicine is that the trust and mandate of the consumer are critical to success. As illustrated by Peters and Waterman, the companies that thrive are those that listen to their customers.

So what communication methods do work for the medical practice? Can public opinion be influenced to counter such negative public sentiment against doctors as that expressed by the 56 percent of those polled by the AMA who believe that doctors are too interested in making money?

There is a growing realization that more and better communication—between doctors and patients, between doctors and medical associations, between doctors and the media, between doctors and the general public—is an important step in the medical profession's ability to recapture the trust, the respect, and the privileges medical practitioners have enjoyed in the past.

Notes
1. Stankaitis, 558. Reprinted by permission from the *New York State Journal of Medicine*, © 1987 by the Medical Society of the State of New York.
2. Owens, 194. Findings taken from *Medical Economics Continuing Survey*. © 1985 by Medical Economics Co., Inc.

2 WHY COMMUNICATE?

For the first time since the Hippocratic oath originated in the fifth century B.C., physicians are threatened by a serious erosion of their authority, prerogative, and status. Long ago, the public's trust was based on a dependence on physicians' knowledge and competence. Trust was founded on family physicians carrying the burden of patient care seven days a week, twenty-four hours a day. It was an earned trust that brought great rewards to the medical profession. Because the public trusted physicians and the public interest was being served, the medical profession was given a relatively free hand to regulate and govern itself. Physicians had their autonomy.

Now the ancient belief that doctors rank just slightly below the Trinity is gone. The new realism sees doctors for what they are, "warts and all," says newspaper editor John Grace.

To some extent, the information explosion and greater education of the public account for the closer public scrutiny of the health care system and its constituents. The media, too, have played a significant role in influencing public sentiment. Intent on exposing wrongdoing, their often negative focus on medical practice has led to a deterioration of trust in doctors.

The price has been high. "This [significant] loss of autonomy is extremely frustrating to doctors. Doctors are pulling their hair out when bureaucrats like me tell them how to practice medicine," Dr. William L. Roper, head of the Medicare program, told the *New York Times*.[1]

A Vote of Approval

American doctors certainly have their admirers. Businessman Richard DeVos, president of Amway Corporation, told Michigan doctors: "You sit around and apologize for your own achievements. You ought to stop it. You should be shouting from the housetops about your accomplishments. You deliver the finest medical care this world has ever seen . . . . With all the talk about 'free' socialized medicine, what you have [in countries with socialized medicine] is a decline in the quality of medicine. The world stands in line to enter this country for medical care."[2]

Opportunities for Communication Overlooked

Why is the American public angry with physicians? Surveys have found that lack of communication is a major problem. Despite the need for taking some initiative, most physicians have remained reticent. Already overextended by their long work hours, they are reluctant to assign a top priority to communicating with the various groups likely to shape the future of health care. They have been slow to educate the public about how biomedical advances are made, why they are costly, and how they might influence lives. Even within the confines of the examining room, many physicians overlook opportunities to cement better relationships with their patients and boost the image of their profession. They have chosen instead to confine their communication to exchanges among themselves, using technical jargon alien to most Americans, says Lawrence Altman of the *New York Times*, a doctor-turned-newsman.

With the exception of the lobbying efforts of organized medical groups attempting to influence local, state, and national government bodies, too little is being done by individual medical practitioners to upgrade the flagging reputation of the profession. Negative press reports and the profession's deteriorating image can be countered by means of a variety of available communication strategies. Dr. Vernon Astler, past president of the Florida Medical Association, states what physicians have frequently been told by their medical associations: "Let us not mistake the battlefield. Human climate and opinion is largely conquered through the ammunition of the communications media . . . . Those of us who remain uninvolved are destined to be governed by those who are involved."[3]

Why Communicate with Patients?

One third of malpractice suits are attributable to ineffective physician-patient communication. For this reason, risk-management strategies often stress developing and enhancing communication skills that create positive interactions with patients. "If doctors spent more time explaining their treatment to their patients, they would probably not wind up in court," says Boston lawyer Steven Rosenthal.

What Every Doctor Should Know: How Patients Grade Physicians

Though the cornerstone of any medical specialty is the clinical ability of the physician, patients use an entirely different measure to evaluate medical services. You may be the finest diagnostician in your area and have impressed your peers, hospital personnel, and medical students on rounds countless times. But how do patients form an estimation of your clinical abilities?

Unable to judge the art of medicine on more than a rudimentary level, most patients base their evaluation on the art of communication. While patients depend on attestations of friends and relatives to a doctor's competence, they respond most strongly to how caring the physician seems and how attentively he or she listens to their complaints. As successful professionals in every field have found, the routine and the normal are not what bring people back, but the extra touch, the unusual. Learning to communicate better with patients reaps many mutually beneficial rewards:

- Patients who feel they have been listened to and understand what the physician says are more likely to trust, to follow treatment regimens, and to be more open about their medical problems, thus facilitating medical care.

- Trusting patients are more likely to refer friends and relatives.

- Medicine can be a more rewarding career when satisfying relationships between doctor and patients can be achieved.

- Fewer malpractice suits are brought against communicative physicians.

Hindrances to Positive Relationships

In the practice of medicine, trust is and always has been dependent on the doctor-patient relationship. However, the reality of the practice of medicine today makes that relationship more difficult to establish and maintain than ever before. It is rapidly deteriorating to a commercial transaction as the focus of health care shifts from relationships based on trust to the marketplace, a shift with profound, pervasive and provocative implications, according to William Kissick, professor of public health and preventive medicine at the University of Pennsylvania.

"There is a growing emphasis on economics and productivity," said Dr. Charles Hatem, director of medical education and associate chief of medicine at Mount Auburn Hospital in Cambridge, Massachusetts. "When you have to bring in so many dollars in so many hours," Dr. Hatem told the press, "it makes good patient relationships impossible."[4]

The altered relationship between doctor and patient often cited in recent years can also be attributed in part to the increasing complexity of medicine and to the resulting shift from general practice to specialization. Some charge that specialists don't know patients, they only know syndromes. Also, medical training does not emphasize caring relationships with patients, nor does society reward these relationships financially. With doctors beginning their practices owing from $40,000 to an estimated $180,000 in education loans, the need to see large numbers of patients is pressing, to the detriment of physician-patient relationships.

The shift to HMOs has also caused changes in the way doctors and patients interact. HMOs have engendered what one physician refers to as a "veterinarian ethic," where primary allegiance is owed not to the patient, but to a third party.

Some physicians predict that as the number of patients enrolling in HMOs increases, fewer families will have the opportunity to establish the types of doctor-patient relationships that engender trust. This could result in unanticipated consequences for those physicians who remain in solo and group practice. While they continue to provide their allegiance directly to their patients, they may be subjected to the general disenchantment with their profession born of generalization.

Patients Still Respect Their Own Physicians

Although the medical profession has experienced some loss of the esteem it once enjoyed, there is a consistent finding in public opinion polls that while most people do not look with favor upon medical practitioners as a group, they continue to respect and support their own personal physicians.

This can be interpreted to mean that once a good relationship develops between patient and physician, it continues to hold the patient's trust. That such bonds with one's own physician no longer seem to generalize to the profession as a whole is among the enigmas now facing medicine.

Communication with Patients Today Is Difficult

Patients, eager for information about health and medicine, have turned to sources other than their physicians for health information. A survey of five hundred physicians by the National Research Corporation, a health care marketing research firm, found that a surprisingly large number of physicians interviewed, 74 percent, said they were not the primary source of medical information for their patients, though approximately 80 percent of physicians noted that their patients were interested in health matters. The author, Joyce Jensen, concluded that if the physician is not his patients' main source of medical information, it is important that he develop adequate lines of communication so patients will discuss their concerns and preferences openly.

The complexity of medicine today presents another problem, according to public relations expert Philip Lesly. "The more any group advances in mastery of its own field, the more certain it is to get out of touch with the rest of the population . . . . In every field, as the subject matter becomes more extensive and complex, two things happen: it requires greater effort by the practitioner to master and keep abreast, and it becomes less understood by outsiders."[5]

Therein lies the challenge. Increased communication is needed at a time when communication is more difficult to achieve.

Counteract Loss of Autonomy with Communication

The medical profession must recapture the primary confidence of the people and maintain and strengthen the public's trust, warned Dr. Walter Judd, a former congressman and member of the AMA's Judicial Council, in 1967; otherwise it risked being converted into a public utility, subject to the sort of regulations imposed on transportation, communications, and power. Indeed, the last twenty-plus years have proven these insightful comments to be prophetic.

Doctors are being treated, in a sense, like any other commodity in the new health care market, which emphasizes competition, efficiency, and stringent controls on costs, Dr. James Todd, deputy executive vice president of the AMA, told the *New York Times*.[6]

How Public Sentiment Leads to Legislation

A 1987 Associated Press article reported that consumer groups were advocating more government control over doctors. The consumers were upset by a "scandalous" jump in physician incomes and "outrageous" physician overcharges for Medicare services, despite the fact that the AMA attributed the rise in income to longer work hours rather than to fee increases.

Dr. Sidney Wolfe, director of the sixty-thousand-member Public Citizen Health Research Group in Washington, D.C., is quoted in the same article as saying that a "public groundswell against high doctor incomes" is developing. Legislation has already been introduced in fifteen states that would force doctors to accept levels of payment set by the government. Such legislation has been enacted in Massachusetts, where, coupled with high malpractice rates and an unfavorable political and economic climate, it has caused doctors to leave that state in search of greater fulfillment elsewhere.

A Cambridge Research Institute poll of public opinion found that 50 percent of respondents strongly favored government price controls and regulations on doctors' fees, with another 27 percent somewhat favoring these measures.[7] In all, an astounding 77 percent of those polled favored government regulation of an industry that has historically been free of such restraints.

The Escalation of Issues

These developments point to the classic pattern of the progress of issues through what has become known as the issue life cycle, which culminates in what business—and that includes the health care business—abhors: government regulation.

The escalation of issues typically begins with unmet public expectations. With what Philip Lesly calls a "sense of entitlement," the public voices social grievances and demands, then forms social action groups which take up the cause. As the public becomes politicized, the media begin to play a major role in the process. The media, by airing grievances, lend a sense of legitimacy to the complaints. If politicized groups don't get satisfaction, they press for legislation. This is precisely the situation in which medicine finds itself as consumers call for more government controls over medical practice.

The Number One Current Issue

Underlying the issue of cost containment is physicians' fear that the quality of care they can deliver will suffer as a result of government regulation of health care costs. Nearly 60 percent of physicians polled by the AMA agreed that quality health care in the United States is threatened by an overemphasis on cost containment.

Donald Cohodes, executive director of policy for Blue Cross and Blue Shield of Chicago, said it is up to physicians "to stand as the protectors of quality in a world lusting for cost containment . . . . If there is an issue lurking on the horizon for the 1990s and beyond, it is quality of care."

Public Must Be Educated about Quality versus Cost

The American public needs to be better informed about the consequences of cost containment and its effect on the medical care they receive.

An extreme preoccupation with cost would entail rationing of care, according to an insurance industry analysis. Some older patients could be denied high-cost procedures. Precise annual maximums on medical payments would be set by insurers, and costs exceeding the limit would be the responsiblity of the patient, which would work in favor of wealthier patients. Medical progress would slow considerably as the pool of funds available for medical research and education dwindled. Medical treatment would be based on statistics, with approval of diagnostic procedures and length of hospital stay based on averages rather than medical judgment. The number of doctors and hospitals would shrink, and patients in some areas would be placed on physicians' waiting lists.

This analysis, presented in the Mercer Meidinger Hansen *Bulletin*, concluded that the social, political, and medical philosophies of the United States would make it unlikely for the above scenario to be played out and that the quality and availability of needed care will continue to take precedence over its cost. Yet while both physicians and the public continue to rate cost as the major problem facing health care, AMA polls indicate that only 21 percent of the public credits doctors with actively trying to hold down the costs of medical care.

The resolution of the quality versus cost controversy depends on two factors: whether a climate of trust in private medicine can be reestablished, and whether costs can be contained sufficiently to allow private medical practice to continue. A climate of trust can be restored only through effective communication.

Effective Communication Offers Substantial Rewards

On both the individual practice and public opinion fronts, how effectively physicians communicate will determine their success and that of their profession. It is generally acknowledged that a particular doctor's image depends less on public perception than on his or her own competence, sense of service, and dedication. In the end, as in the beginning, we come full circle to the importance of the doctor-patient relationship. How these relationships are managed will determine whether medical practices grow and prosper. The trust built by those relationships begets a better image for the profession and mitigates against the expectation of wrongdoing by doctors, thereby decreasing the push toward government regulation.

The American public's response to the health care delivery system is influenced by sources both inside and outside the system. These include patients, physicians, government, the media, alternative delivery systems such as HMOs and PPOs, business groups, and others seeking to change the way health care is organized, delivered, and reimbursed. All are using their influence to shape the delivery of health care. Individually and collectively, the medical profession can and should exert its considerable influence to shape the future. The tool is communication. The target is public opinion. The payoff is survival of fee-for-service medical practice.

Notes
1. *See* Pear, 10.
2. Weddon, 562.
3. Astler, 566.
4. *See* Okrent, 92.
5. *See* Welton, 153.
6. *See* note 1.
7. Shapiro and Young, 410.

Part II

CONSERVATIVE COMMUNICATION STRATEGIES

Effective communication can be achieved in a variety of ways. Comprehensive communication programs are multifaceted and often include several of the following elements:

- Strengthening and maximizing communication effectiveness with current and potential patients

- Developing practical communication aids such as patient information publications, medical newsletters, and audiovisual materials

- Participating in speakers bureaus, community seminars, and professional forums

- Aiding and supplementing efforts of organized medical associations

- Identifying and working with the opinion makers and lawmakers who influence the course of health care delivery in this country

- Establishing good working relations with the media on both the local and national levels

Communication activities can vary widely along a conservative-aggressive continuum. Those activities considered most conservative are confined to relations between a practice and its patients.

In general, the aim is to improve the quality of the interactions between physicians, their staff, and patients. Such activities do not raise eyebrows among colleagues and can dramatically increase patient satisfaction. A sound patient-relations program is the backbone of any communications effort, and the measures taken to improve communication with patients, if given priority, benefit the practice, the patients, and the medical profession. Since most medical specialties depend on word-of-mouth referrals for their continued well-being, improved communication with patients is well worth the effort, according to those who have learned what it takes to attract patients and to keep them.

Conservative communication approaches include efforts to educate patients about their illness, about health, and to inform them about your practice, specialty, and other related matters. Programs remain within the conservative communication category when health education materials are distributed to current patients. Patient education programs can also gain community recognition for a practice.

The three arenas for implementing these strategies are physician-patient relations, office staff-patient interactions, and the physical office setting. There are also three opportunities to enhance interactions: prior to, during, and after patient visits.

Physicians have reported that many of the conservative measures covered in Part II are effective, often cost-free practice enhancers.

3 PRACTICE ASSESSMENT

Know your patients, your service area, and your competition. That advice is given by virtually every consultant to physicians considering any communication effort, no matter how small or large in scope. Many consultants also advise that each member of a practice consider his or her own goals, both personal and professional, prior to making any change.

Practice assessment determines the health of a practice, gives direction to plans for any needed or desired changes, and provides valuable information about the practice and the practice area. Practice assessment answers such questions as:

Who are our current patients?

What are their demographic characteristics?

Are they clustered in any particular geographic location?

How do they perceive the practice?

Who are potential new patients?

Where are they located?

Who else in the area can provide their medical care?

What types of patients does our practice best serve?

Are these the patients currently being served?

Do we want to make any changes in the practice to better suit our lifestyle and professional goals?

How and by whom are patients referred to the practice?

Practice analysis is a somewhat time-consuming process, but, like the complete history and physical at the first visit, it is essential. Gathering information about the practice, the practice area, and the practitioners is well worth the time, effort, and any cost incurred in this initial phase of the communication process. In the long run, basing a communication or career strategy on a solid footing saves time, money and energy.

Know Your Patients

Begin the practice assessment by obtaining a *demographic profile* of patients in the practice: age, income level, occupation, marital status, insurance coverage, address (by zip code), and ethnic, cultural, or language background. Use the forms illustrated opposite to collect and organize demographic information from office records. If your office is equipped with a computerized billing system, your computer may be able to sort patients by some of their characteristics. Consult your manual or your software company's support personnel to determine whether such reports can be generated.

Determine the *demographic profile of the practice area*, especially if you wish to increase the number of patients in your practice. Look for significant shifts in popula-

PATIENT ANALYSIS FORM -- BY AGE

	MALE		FEMALE		TOTAL	
AGE	number	%	number	%	number	%
0-18*						
19-44						
45-64						
65+						

* Change to 5- or 10-year intervals if age is an important factor in the practice.

PATIENT ANALYSIS FORM -- BY ETHNIC/LANGUAGE BACKGROUND

	number	% of practice
White*		
Black		
Hispanic		
Asian		
Other nonwhite		

* Use more refined breakdown, e.g., Polish-American, Irish-American, if it would provide more useful information to the practice.

PATIENT ANALYSIS FORM -- BY INSURANCE CARRIER

INSURER	number	% of practice
Medicare		
Medicaid		
Blue Shield		
Other private		
HMO		
Self-pay		

tion, age, sex, and income levels in the community. This analysis will answer such questions as: Is it time to open a satellite office, or to change location altogether? Are there potential patients who could be well served but who may be unaware the practice is available? Much of this information may be available from marketing departments of local hospitals, the local library, or the Chamber of Commerce. County or state medical societies may also be able to provide area demographic information.

Occupational data is also valuable. Find out how many patients and how much of the practice's revenue are represented by major area employers, particularly since many firms have become buyers of physician services and may contact a physician directly to negotiate discounted fees.

Practices lacking the time and personnel to collect demographic data can commission a customized patient and practice area demographic study from marketing and public relations consultants (see chapter 14, "Hiring a Consultant"), or from the American Medical Association's Department of Practice Management in Chicago, which can be contacted at (312) 645-5000.

Greg Korneluk, a well-known practice-management consultant, recommends a *telephone census* to accurately determine the number of active patients. Hire college students or part-time assistants for approximately a week's time, which should prove sufficient to complete phoning the entire patient roster. Give callers a script (see opposite). Instruct them to tell patients they're calling to update your files, then ask questions about any changes in name, address, employment, and insurance.

Questioning will determine whether the patient is still active. Repeat the census twice a year. If it shows that more patients are coming in than going out, the practice is reasonably healthy.

SAMPLE TELEPHONE CENSUS FORM

Patient Name_______________________________
Patient Number__________Date Called_________
Caller initials____

"Hello. My name is _________________ and I'm calling for Dr.______________. We are currently updating the information in our patient files and would like to know whether the following is still accurate:"

If patient is female, ask, "Is your last name still _________________?" (If necessary, say, "Sometimes people's names change when they get married.")

"Are you still living at ______?" (give address: street, city, state, ZIP code)

"Are you still covered by (name of insurance carrier) ________?"

"The identification number we have is __________. Is that correct?"

If the patient indicates that he or she is no longer the doctor's patient, ask, "Would you mind telling me the reasons you no longer see Dr.___?"

Reason(s) for leaving:

If the patient has moved, ask, "How far is that from your former address?" _____________

If the patient expresses dissatisfaction, ask, "With the physician or the office staff?"

Pursue with "What happened?"

End with "Thank you for your time."

Determine Patient Attitudes and Opinions

A patient questionnaire provides a wealth of information about practice-related issues. It can be used to assess patient opinions of the physician(s) and staff, whether patients understand the specialty, what they think of the physical facility and its location, and whether they are satisfied with the health information they receive.

Its purpose is not only to determine what patients think of the practice, but also to point out what changes might better satisfy patients.

Questionnaires can be administered in a number of ways. In the initial practice assessment phase, questionnaires are used as a research tool. Typically, one hundred questionnaires are mailed to a randomly selected sample of patients to determine specific problems and to gauge strengths and weaknesses of the practice. It is not necessary to poll all patients. A cover letter asks patients to fill out the questionnaire and mail it back. Postage is customarily prepaid.

When the questionnaires are returned, results are tabulated and presented to the doctor. As an alternative to mailing, questionnaires can be given to office patients over a period of a week or two or until one hundred have been completed.

Several months after analysis of the initial questionnaires is completed, the entire questionnaire or specific portions of it can again be administered, in the office, either periodically or on an ongoing basis. This is done to elicit patient feedback, to determine whether problems have been corrected, and to keep the communication effort on track.

The sample questionnaire below covers ten areas of medical practice in which potential problems can be identified and remedied. It can be used in whole or in part.

PATIENT QUESTIONNAIRE

Below are statements with which you may strongly agree, strongly disagree, or in between. Please check the box that most closely reflects your experience. We would also appreciate any suggestions you may have. Space is provided at the end of each section for your suggestions.

I. APPOINTMENTS	Strongly agree				Strongly disagree
1. When I called for an appointment, I received one within an acceptable time frame.	☐	☐	☐	☐	☐
2. The receptionist was helpful in setting up an appointment.	☐	☐	☐	☐	☐
3. I find available appointment times convenient. (If not, please indicate what you would consider convenient office hours: (____________)	☐	☐	☐	☐	☐
4. The receptionist was courteous.	☐	☐	☐	☐	☐

Suggestions:

II. OFFICE VISIT	Strongly agree				Strongly disagree
5. When I arrived at the office, I was greeted in a friendly manner.	☐	☐	☐	☐	☐
6. The waiting time to see the doctor was reasonable. I waited ___________ minutes.	☐	☐	☐	☐	☐
7. The surroundings were neat and attractive.	☐	☐	☐	☐	☐
8. The waiting room furniture was comfortable.	☐	☐	☐	☐	☐
9. Reading materials in the waiting room were of interest to me.	☐	☐	☐	☐	☐

Suggestions:

III. LOCATION

10. The office location is convenient for me.	☐	☐	☐	☐	☐
11. Parking or transportation were easy to find.	☐	☐	☐	☐	☐
12. It takes a reasonable amount of time for me to get to the office. (Please note how long: _______ min.)	☐	☐	☐	☐	☐

Suggestions:

IV. ANCILLARY OFFICE STAFF

	Strongly agree				Strongly disagree
13. The nurse meets my needs.	☐	☐	☐	☐	☐
14. Office staff are available and willing to answer any questions I have.	☐	☐	☐	☐	☐
15. My privacy is respected.	☐	☐	☐	☐	☐
16. I am familiar with office billing and payment policies.	☐	☐	☐	☐	☐
17. These policies were explained to me well. (By whom?____________________)	☐	☐	☐	☐	☐
18. I am satisfied with the arrangement this office has for filing insurance claims.	☐	☐	☐	☐	☐

Suggestions:

V. QUALITY OF CARE

19. I feel I was evaluated thoroughly by the doctor.	☐	☐	☐	☐	☐
20. I feel the physician's care achieved the desired results in a reasonable amount of time.	☐	☐	☐	☐	☐
21. I feel I received quality service. (If not, how could it be improved?)	☐	☐	☐	☐	☐

Suggestions:

VI. PHYSICIAN

	Strongly agree				Strongly disagree
22. The doctor's manner is excellent.	☐	☐	☐	☐	☐
23. I feel confident in the doctor.	☐	☐	☐	☐	☐
24. The doctor spends enough time with me.	☐	☐	☐	☐	☐
25. I have ample opportunity to explain to the doctor what is bothering me.	☐	☐	☐	☐	☐
26. The doctor listens to my concerns.	☐	☐	☐	☐	☐
27. The doctor fully explained my condition.	☐	☐	☐	☐	☐
28. The doctor fully explained the treatment.	☐	☐	☐	☐	☐

Was there anything you didn't understand when you left the office? If yes, what was it, and how did you get an answer?

Suggestions:

VII. FEES

	Strongly agree				Strongly disagree
29. In my estimation, fees are competitive and reasonable.	☐	☐	☐	☐	☐
30. My insurance covers most or all of my medical bills.	☐	☐	☐	☐	☐

Suggestions:

VIII. BILLS

31. I receive statements in a timely fashion.	☐	☐	☐	☐	☐
32. The format of the bills is easy to understand.	☐	☐	☐	☐	☐
33. If I have questions about the bill, the staff answers them to my satisfaction.	☐	☐	☐	☐	☐

Suggestions:

IX. DELINQUENT ACCOUNTS

If our office has had occasion to contact you regarding a delinquent account, please answer the next two questions.

34. I found the contact to be professional.	☐	☐	☐	☐	☐

	Strongly agree				Strongly disagree
35. I responded favorably.	☐	☐	☐	☐	☐

Suggestions:

X. ANSWERING SERVICE; COVERAGE

Reply only if you have had occasion to deal with the answering service and/or other doctors covering the practice.

36. Answering service personnel are courteous.	☐	☐	☐	☐	☐
37. The answering service relayed my message to the doctor promptly.	☐	☐	☐	☐	☐
38. The physician(s) who cover the doctor's practice are courteous.(I was seen by Dr.________________________)	☐	☐	☐	☐	☐
39. The covering physician was familiar with my condition and had access to my records.	☐	☐	☐	☐	☐
40. The covering doctor provided care comparable in quality to the care I receive from my regular physician.	☐	☐	☐	☐	☐

Suggestions:

Another good source of information about patient attitudes and opinions is office staff, who work with patients on a daily basis. Useful insights can be gained by asking staff what they think patients like and don't like about the practice. However, a more accurate way to monitor patient satisfaction is to provide a log book and ask secretaries, receptionists, nurses, and billing personnel to log all patient complaints and compliments.

Determine Why Patients Leave

If desirable patients are deserting the practice, it is important to find out why. Patients have many reasons for leaving, some that can be remedied and others, like a patient moving out of state, that are unrelated to the practice. Call patients who have left the practice and tabulate information on their reasons for doing so. Use the chart on page 40 to track their replies, and whether additional patients leave after measures are taken to remedy practice-related problems.

Know Your Referral Sources

This information forms the basis of any communication plan. You may opt to use communication efforts to maximize referrals from colleagues, to focus on existing and potential patients, or to combine these. However, you cannot determine how much effort should go into each source until you have a clear idea of how new patients are currently coming into the practice.

To obtain this information (see chart, page 41), ask new patients who referred them and how they heard about the practice. Keep a separate listing of which physicians refer patients, and how many they refer.

Staff and Office Assessment

It is far less expensive to keep patients you already have than to attract new ones, and consultants advise getting your house in order before spending any money on communication activities. Office ambiance, not

PATIENTS LEAVING ANALYSIS

Period covered: January 1 to June 30, 1990

Total patients leaving ________

Total new patients ________

Reasons for Leaving

1. Moved (more than 10 miles) ________

2. Moved (less than 10 miles) ________

3. Doesn't want treatment ________

4. Dissatisfaction with physician ________

   Dr. A ________
   Dr. B ________
   Dr. C ________

5. Dissatisfaction with office staff ________

   Office Manager ________
   Receptionist ________
   Nurse ________
   Billing personnel ________
   Other ________

6. Requests for payment at time of service ________

7. Other (specify) ________

8. Patients dismissed for non-compliance with office policies ________

medical expertise, is what most often attracts patients. The majority of patients view medical services by doctors in a particular specialty as similar. Patients, who generally cannot judge medical expertise, base their choices on factors more tangible to them, including staff courtesy, physician's manner, convenience of location, and waiting time for appointments.

PATIENT REFERRAL REPORT

New Patient Referral Sources

	Jan	Feb	Mar	Apr	May	Jun	Jul	Aug	Sep	Oct	Nov	Dec
Patients												
MDs												
Hospital A												
Hospital B												
Emergency Room A												
Emergency Room B												
Telephone Directory												
Walk-ins												
Industry												
Schools												
Community Activities												
Lectures												
Radio, TV												
Newspaper												
Promotion A												
Promotion B												
Other												

The two most common methods for assessing medical office staff are direct observation and patient questionnaires (see Patient Questionnaire, staff portion). Consultants advise physicians to use other means of determining their staffs' interactions with patients as well. They suggest paying close attention to patients' comments about employees, even those seemingly said in jest.

It may also be useful for a physician to phone the office number from time to time to see how long it takes before the phone is answered and to note the tone of voice that comes across.

Self Assessment and Practice Assessment

Self Assessment

Each physician in the practice should rate his or her own interpersonal skills, major strengths and weaknesses, satisfaction with the types of patients being seen, and personal goals and ambitions. Each member of a group practice should conduct this type of assessment. An assessment for the group as a whole should be conducted as well.

Practice Assessment

Delineating practice goals and objectives gives shape to the future of the practice. Such factors as patient load, desired income, ethical, professional, and personal goals need to be considered. Goals are the ends toward which your efforts will be directed. Is the goal to increase patient load? Increase income? Attract a different group of patients? Increase free time? Change the practice so that it will yield a more rewarding career? Improve retention rate of current patients? Increase referrals? Spell out goals as briefly and as specifically as possible.

SELF AND PRACTICE ASSESSMENT

This practice's greatest strengths are:

1. ______________________

2. ______________________

3. ______________________

The greatest strengths I bring to this practice are:

1. ______________________

2. ______________________

3. ______________________

This practice's greatest weaknesses are:

1. ______________________

2. ______________________

3. ______________________

The following in my relationships with my patients could improve:

1. ______________________

2. ______________________

3. ______________________

4. ______________________

The following in my relationships with my partners could improve:

1. ______________________________

2. ______________________________

3. ______________________________

The patients I most enjoy treating have the following basic characteristics:

1. ______________________________

2. ______________________________

3. ______________________________

4. ______________________________

The patients who have these characteristics represent approximately _______ percent of the patients I am now seeing.

This practice's professional and business goals are:

1. ______________________________

2. ______________________________

3. ______________________________

4. ______________________________

The following are my own professional goals:

1. ______________________________

2. ______________________________

3. ______________________________

On a scale of 1 to 10, the professional and business goals listed above coincide _____ with my own professional and business goals.

The primary personal goals and ambitions I hope to realize through the practice of medicine are:

1. ______________________________

2. ______________________________

3. ______________________________

Your goals will be met by stating objectives to be reached in a specified time period. If the goal is to increase patient load, the objective might be to attract 25 new patients per month or to increase the load of patients with gastrointestinal complaints by 25 percent in the next six months.

To determine whether goals can be achieved, information about the current patient base, referral sources, the competition, patient decision-making processes, and the strengths and weaknesses of the practice is needed. It is also useful to note whether there is something about the practice that gives it a competitive edge and, if so, whether it could attract patients whose health problems the practice is best at handling without narrowing the patient base too much.

In a group practice, it is important to have consensus on the direction the practice should take before any planning takes place, lest the process be undermined in the implementation phase. If one member of the group is so opposed to the plan that he or she cannot support it, perhaps that person's withrawal from the practice would serve the group best, according to consultants Leif Beck, Geoffrey Anders, and Dorothy Sweeney.

Consultants also advise assessing the range of services offered, and determining whether other services could be provided to move the practice in the desired direction. If new services are to be added, it is important to have as much information as is available on the competition, and to assess the impact on referrals. A pulmonary specialist whose practice is largely dependent on referrals may see those referrals dry up if he decides to enlarge his practice to include general internal medicine.

Know Your Practice Area

Identify and assess the competition.

Do other physicians, HMOs, walk-in centers, non-physician providers, or hospital facilities compete with the practice for patients? What are each competitor's strengths, weaknesses, and future plans?

Questions to ask:

What services do others offer, and how do these services compare with those of our own practice?

Does the competition have advantages in technology, resources, personnel, convenience, price, public perception, or quality?

To which patients are these advantages likely to appeal?

Can we compete effectively for these patients, and should we?

What distinguishes our practice from that of competitors?

How can we use our advantages to maximize patient load or patient satisfaction?

What, if any, marketing strategies and target markets are competitors pursuing?

What are our competitors' future plans?

Information on local competitors can be obtained from state and county medical societies and the AMA's Market Area Profile (MAP) service, established to provide precisely this type of information. Competitors' future plans can be gleaned from gossip, rumors, and lunchtime conversations at the hospital cafeteria. Don't underestimate the grapevine as a source of valuable information.

Area demographics, including assessment of the local business and economic environment, can also provide valuable information to a medical practice. Gather facts on employment trends, businesses moving into the area, and the presence of industries that might affect disease incidence.

Such information is available from the AMA, from county planning commissions, from business groups, including the Chamber of Commerce, and from state and county medical associations.

Other service-area factors that might impact on the practice include physical and psychological parameters. *Physical parameters* are such natural boundaries as lakes, mountains, and rivers, or major land use zones, including airports and industrial parks. *Psychological parameters* include such barriers as "wrong side of the tracks." This concept might either discourage people from seeking services in one part of town or encourage them to favor a certain area. Practices in communities close to, yet outside of, major metropolitan areas are often snubbed because people perceive that better medical care is available "in town." Such prejudices can be overcome if their existence is known.

4 HOW TO SATISFY PATIENTS: OFFICE STRATEGIES

The first step in planning and implementing a communication strategy involves making desired changes in your facility and in office policies and procedures. Many of the problem areas related to the office, identified during the practice assessment, can be quickly remedied. Staff awareness of problem areas, coupled with a bit of advice and a few pats on the back, are often sufficient to create the type of patient-oriented office that contributes to a thriving practice.

A comfortable and convenient office, a courteous staff, and patient-oriented policies and procedures encourage a favorable image of the practice and communicate to patients a caring, healing environment, even before they meet the doctor.

How Patients Choose a Physician

Researchers Crane and Lynch found that the two most important criteria used by consumers to choose a physician are competence and courtesy.[1]

However, because prospective patients cannot experience these directly before visiting a physician, they form perceptions about the practice from secondhand cues: from referrals, from the location of the office, and from communication, direct and indirect, emanating from the physician's office. A physician who locates his or her office in a prestigious area, who sends a practice brochure, and whose knowledgeable staff takes the time to provide all necessary information to a patient, conveys a quality image.

At the time of the first appointment, initial expectations, derived from these secondary cues, will be positively or negatively reinforced. Then, the tenor of the visit determines whether the patient will return.

Patients: What They Want and How to Keep Them

First Impressions

A patient's first impressions are formed by the courtesy with which he or she is greeted by the receptionist, and the location and appearance of the office. The type of building, the furniture, and the clientele are all important cues patients use to assess "competence."

Studies have found that the office is the second most important cue, after personal referral, in the selection of a physician. Not only the look of the office, but the appearance and the number of other patients in the waiting room make important first impressions that serve as indicators of competence. Patients expect to see others in a doctor's waiting room, and they form some of their perceptions of the practice by observing those who are waiting.

The Office

Locate your office relatively close to the patients you wish to attract. If, through the patient questionnaire, you find that a significant number of patients spend thirty minutes traveling to your office, ask yourself, "If another physician in the same specialty opened an office ten minutes from these patients tomorrow, how many patients would I lose?" Perhaps it is time to open a satellite office, or to relocate. A pediatrician would be well advised to relocate his practice from an aging community to one with an influx of young families. A plastic surgeon, on the other hand, may want to open a satellite office convenient to a middle-aged, affluent population. Such major and costly undertakings should be implemented only after a careful demographic assessment, like the one provided by the American Medical Association's MAP program.

Assess your physical facility based on the following advice from practice management consultants:

> If you lease your office, insist that the building be kept clean and in good repair.
>
> Parking should be easily accessible. If older patients comprise a large part of your practice, it may help to be on a public transportation line.
>
> The office should be large enough for comfort and efficiency, clean and fresh looking.
>
> Privacy should be afforded for discussion of fees and financial arrangements, and for telephone conversations with patients.
>
> When decorating the office, remember that many health care decisions are made by women—for themselves, their spouses, and their children. Make sure your decor appeals to both sexes—many medical offices are decorated to appeal primarily to men.
>
> Display diplomas, awards, and newspaper clips about your practice in your office and reception area. For a more personal look, display pictures of your family.

Furnish the waiting room with chairs rather than couches: most people don't like to sit close to strangers, particularly when they are not feeling well.

Fresh flowers and holiday decorations in the waiting room can help put patients at ease. Some consultants advocate soft, relaxing music to create a pleasant atmosphere.

If children are frequent visitors, design a children's corner with games, puzzles, and coloring books to keep them busy and away from older patients.

Choose reading materials that are of interest to your patients—not just those you like to read.

Begin an office library. Provide books, pamphlets, brochures, and audiovisual materials related to your specialty that can be circulated among your patients.

Consider displaying the work of local artists in your reception area. Art displays make your office more attractive and give exposure to the artist.

Make available brochures about local attractions, travel, and entertainment—especially if many of your patients come from out of town in order to take advantage of your specialty.

The Examining Room

Examining rooms should be neat, clean, bright, and cheerful. Furnish them with magazines, brochures, or other reading matter for patients who are kept waiting.

Assure patients privacy. If you must leave the room to consult with another patient or a staff member, make sure to close the door behind you.

Keep the temperature in the exam room comfortable for those who are undressed.

You and Your Staff

The way members of your staff communicate with patients can be just as important to your practice as your own communication with patients. A marginal staff can be a physician's worst enemy, says practice management specialist Gregory Korneluk. Indeed, a study by Donald Christensen and Thomas Giese found friendliness of the receptionist to be the most important indicator of patient satisfaction. Programs to train staff in patient relations are available from many hospitals, medical societies, and consultants. The programs focus on improving staff courtesy, telephone manner, and handling of billing problems.

Consultants offer the following tips for maximizing office staff-patient interactions, designed to make your staff an important part of your communication efforts:

Insist that your staff be courteous to patients. When problems arise, whether they be billing problems, missed appointments, or too frequent calls to the physician, instruct the staff to give the patient the benefit of the doubt.

Set a good example: behave toward patients as you would like your staff to behave.

When hiring new staff, give as much weight to their attitude and friendliness as to their professional skills.

Hold regular staff meetings to discuss patient relations and to involve staff members in your communication objectives, or hire a consultant to provide patient relations training to your office staff.

Discuss problems (for example, rudeness, keeping patients on hold too long) with staff members. Give staff the opportunity to correct their behavior before issuing a formal warning or considering dismissal.

Compliment staff members who perform well with a "good job" or an appreciative note.

Instruct your staff to offer to help patients with their insurance forms, particularly if they have repeated problems with them.

Reward staff for special projects or objectives completed with a day off or a cash bonus.

If you keep evening or Saturday hours, allow your staff time off during the week for shopping or personal time. Hire part-time workers to fill any gaps.

Take advantage of flextime and staggered lunch hours to cover early morning or evening hours. Some staff prefer a 7:00 a.m.–3:00 p.m. shift, which accommodates patients who like to come in before work. Others may prefer working from noon to 8:00 p.m., or evenings and Saturdays only.

Inform the office staff of the availability of written information, classes, and support groups provided by local and state hospitals, and medical and community organizations. In the absence of a patient newsletter, instruct your staff to inform appropriate patients of these additional resources.

Staff and Patients

Staff should be taught to observe the following niceties:

Because patients hate excessive waiting times for appointments most, acknowledge any delays immediately. If possible, call patients before they leave for the office. Tell those in the waiting room why the doctor has been delayed, and approximately how long the delay will be.

When a patient asks a staff member a question he or she cannot answer, the best response is "I don't know, but I'll be happy to find out for you." Then follow up.

Be on the alert for any patient dissatisfaction and attempt to clarify any misunderstanding.

Answer the telephone with a friendly voice, and when you have to put calls on hold, try to do it for no longer than thirty seconds.

Give callers an estimated time within which the doctor will return their call. Letting patients know that "the doctor usually returns calls after 5:30 p.m" frees them from lengthy periods of waiting for the call.

In an emergency, provide reassurance by letting the patient know you will make every effort to reach the doctor in the next few minutes.

Remain calm with callers who are angry or upset. Convey factual information about what is being done to resolve a matter as promptly as possible.

Scheduling

The following suggestions were made by the Department of Communications and Physician Marketing of the Ohio State Medical Association:

Don't let your staff overbook your schedule.

Have your staff verify office appointments by phone, and, if you so desire, rearrange your schedule if you have a number of cancellations.

Set aside time each day for new patients, walk-ins or emergencies so that such occurrences do not disrupt your schedule.

Consider alternating office hours each day to accommodate varying patient schedules. This often works to keep staff happy, too.

Offer evening and weekend appointments for working patients or those whose schedules make it difficult to see you during the daytime. If this is not possible, set aside the first and last appointments of the day for these patients.

If your office is located in or near a shopping area and the wait to see you will be long, provide your patients with a beeper so they can leave and go shopping nearby.

Collections

Many physicians prefer to let their office staff take care of the touchy matter of unpaid bills. However, as more and more attention is being drawn to the high cost of health care, and as more patients ask questions about charges for care, physicians have to become comfortable discussing fees. What's more, too many delinquent accounts can have a serious impact on your ability to continue practicing medicine.

The following are some tips for avoiding problems with collections and for handling problems once they occur:

Make a written fee schedule available to patients upon request, so that they know in advance what certain procedures will cost and what insurance is likely to cover. A geriatric practitioner, for example, might add a statement at the bottom of the fee schedule informing patients that Medicare pays 80 percent of the amount approved, and that the patient or his coinsurer is responsible for the other 20 percent.

Encourage patients to check with their insurance companies so that they know which procedures are and are not going to be covered, and what their deductible and copayment responsibilities will be.

State your payment policies. Post a notice about your policies in the waiting room and on the receptionist's desk. Have your staff explain the payment policies to new patients at the time of their first visit, and include payment information on appropriate written communication to your patients. A typical notice might read as follows:

> **PAYMENT IS EXPECTED**
> **WHEN SERVICES ARE RENDERED**
> **UNLESS OTHER ARRANGEMENTS**
> **ARE MADE IN ADVANCE.**
>
> **THANK YOU.**

When possible, request payment at the time of the visit. It is easier for the receptionist to make the request at that time if the policy is stated in writing. For insured patients, request an insurance form if your office completes them or, if patients submit their own forms, ask that they complete the form prior to leaving the office.

Payment Plans

Encourage patients to discuss any financial problems they may have, and attempt to work out an affordable payment plan with patients who are having such difficulties.

If the patient misses more than one or two payments, stress that you expect a good-faith effort by the patient to pay something monthly, even if it is less than the agreed upon amount.

Delinquent Accounts

When first approaching a delinquent account, ask if the patient is experiencing financial difficulties, and if there is any way you can be of assistance. Make it clear that you value and want to keep the patient.

Collection Letters

Collection letters should be signed by the office manager. Handwritten personal notes are often effective in convincing a patient to pay a bill. As a last resort, a personal note from the physician may help make a patient feel obligated to pay (see example opposite).

Insurance Forms

Make sure that your office staff is adequately trained to provide assistance to patients in completing their insurance forms. Many practices complete and submit forms for their patients, after the patients fill out their portion of the claim form.

When appropriate, ask patients to sign direct authorization of payments to you. This avoids delays and misunderstandings on what the patient owes and what the insurance company will pay.

Collection Agency versus Discount

A note on a bill stating, "If no payment is received by *[date]*, this account will be turned over to collections" often elicits payment.

Collection agencies charge 30 percent to 50 percent of proceeds they collect. Before handing over an account, consider offering the patient a 10 percent or 20 percent discount for immediate payment.

Don't Delay Action on Delinquent Accounts

The more time goes by, the less likely the patient is to feel obligated to pay a bill. Contact patients about unpaid accounts after a set time, usually 90 days.

Telephone Tips

Consider reserving a time each day for patients to call you with their health care concerns, but only if the nature of your practice allows you to be there daily during that time.

Don't keep patients who call on hold too long. If patients consistently have to hold for a minute or more because the secretary is busy answering other calls, it may be a signal that your practice has grown to the

Mr. John H. Smith
123 Main St.
Anywhere, US 12345

Re: Account #4861

Dear Mr. Smith:

As you know, your account with us is now long overdue. We realize that medical expenses can sometimes impose unexpected financial problems. Often it seems that such problems are dealt with impersonally. I'm sorry if it seems that way.

If a mistake has been made in the processing of your account, please give us the opportunity to correct it. If you have simply overlooked this matter, please send us your check today, along with this letter, in the enclosed envelope.

If, however, your circumstances are such that you cannot pay immediately, or if you are unable to make full payment, it is essential that you write a short explanatory note on the reverse side of this letter and return it to us today. It certainly is not our desire to turn your overdue account to [a collection agency, our collections staff, our lawyer]. We hate to do it, but if you do not contact us promptly by mail or telephone, we will be forced to assign this account to our [collection agency, collections staff, lawyer] in ten days.

Sincerely,

[Office Manager or Billing Department, William S. Brown, M.D.]

If two or more addresses appear on your letterhead, add the following to the end of the letter:

PLEASE RESPOND TO (NAME OF TOWN) ADDRESS

point of your having to hire a second receptionist.

Monitor busy signals. Ask the telephone company to monitor your line to determine how many callers get busy signals when they call your office, and the time of day your office gets the most phone calls. Better scheduling of staff, or adding call waiting or a second telephone line may be indicated.

If you use an answering machine when you are not in the office, make sure your message makes it clear how you can be reached in an emergency or who is covering for you in your absence. Check the answering machine regularly to make sure it is in good working order.

If you employ an answering service, check periodically to make sure it is providing quality service.

If calls to your office from a neighboring community are subject to long-distance charges, consider putting in a toll-free number or a local line.

Use the Mail

Mailings provide another good way to keep in touch with patients. They are widely used by physicians for the following purposes:

> Send postcards to remind patients of appointments, especially those scheduled more than a month in advance. Postcards can also be used to remind patients of check-ups, immunizations, annual physicals, and so on.
>
> Mark occasions by sending holiday and birthday cards to your regular patients.
>
> Printed sympathy cards or personal notes may be sent to relatives of deceased patients to express sympathy. Dr. John Erhardt of Salt Lake City relates that his brief note to the family of a deceased

patient, stating his sincere feelings that it was an honor and a privilege to have been chosen as that person's physician, was truly appreciated by the family. If appropriate, flowers or a personal visit may be in order.

Gifts

Some consultants advocate giving small gifts to patients. Their suggestions include:

Small items or coupons for those who have to wait more than fifteen minutes to see you.

Folders with your practice name and logo in which they can keep their records, receipts, appointment cards, health information sheets, and brochures.

Gifts such as T-shirts with your office logo, carrying bags, medical travel kits, first-aid kits, to let patients know how much you value their patronage.

Flowers for patients who have referred a new patient to you.

Solicit Patient Feedback

Patient follow-up through solicitation of comments, suggestions, and complaints helps keep your staff on their toes and lets patients know you care.

Use patient questionnaires (see chapter 3).

A phone call to patients who have left the practice may uncover problems and provide valuable feedback. Try to find out why they switched to another provider.

Install a suggestion box in the reception area and provide paper and pens to solicit patient complaints, concerns—and compliments. Keep a list of patient complaints, both written and verbal, in a ledger, and tally them periodically. If complaints fall into one area, for example, "waiting time is too long," take steps to remedy the situation.

Notes
1. Crane and Lynch, 17. Reprinted from *Journal of Health Care Marketing*, 1988, Vol. 8, No. 3, published by the American Marketing Association.

5 MAKING THE MOST OF THE VISIT: EFFECTIVE DOCTOR-PATIENT COMMUNICATION

Patients' number one complaint is that physicians don't spend enough time with them, Robert B. Doherty, a spokesman for the American Society of Internal Medicine, told the *Wall Street Journal.*[1] They want and are demanding what they perceive to be quality medical care—a doctor skilled in communication as well as clinical skills, who knows how to satisfy patients and make the time spent with them count. Success in retaining current patients and attracting new ones is the key to a thriving practice, and patient willingness to remain with any individual provider depends on the patient's level of satisfaction with that doctor. Physicians have found that it works both ways: satisfying relationships with patients are a source of intrinsic reward and an important factor in their own job satisfaction.

Medical society and risk-management literature consistently stresses communication with patients as among the most effective means of avoiding malpractice lawsuits. Yet in the 1987 AMA public opinion poll, the last time the question was asked, only 45 percent of respondents agreed that "Doctors usually explain things well to their patients," down from 55 percent in 1982.

When asked what they want of their physicians, patients respond most frequently that they want enhanced communication, according to research by health care marketing authority Robin MacStravic, and Joyce Jensen of the National Research Corporation.

MacStravic's survey of four hundred patients revealed that eleven factors comprise the tangible evidence patients use as their basis for feeling satisfied with a doctor.[2] They are, in order of importance:

- Taking time/being thorough
- Explaining procedures thoroughly
- Showing interest beyond the immediate problem
- Using understandable language
- Getting good results
- Being straightforward, honest, and open
- Being available when needed
- Being confident, assured
- Following up, checking on patients
- Listening, being attentive
- Answering questions

Certain attributes carry more weight than others. Patients will endure personal physicians whose offices are inconveniently located, who are often unavailable, and who charge too much. But they will not tolerate physicians they perceive to be uncaring, incompetent, and unfriendly.

A review of sixty studies of doctor-patient interviews found that the strongest predictor of patient satisfaction with a physician is the amount of information the doctor gives about the patient's condition and its treatment. Specifically, patients want basic information:

- A diagnosis. What is wrong?
- A cause. Why do I have this condition?
- A treatment plan. What should be done about it? Are there options? What are they? What side effects are associated with each?
- Outcome. Will I recover? How long will it take?
- Cost. How much will the treatment cost? Will my insurance cover it?

Unless these questions are answered in understandable terms, the patient will leave the office dissatisfied. And as long as they receive the type of care they need and want, patients will not be angered by physicians' high income, a Baltimore medical society committee concluded after its survey of public opinion.

The Effective Medical Interview

Clearly, the key to patient satisfaction is the physician's ability and willingness to communicate. Yet effective communication with patients is apparently not taught in medical schools. Interviewing is a case in point. "Like many human basics—parenting, teaching, sex—the medical interview is seldom taught, or studied, even by those who do it often," according to Dr. Mack Lipkin, Jr., director of the National Task Force on Medical Interviews.[3] He told the *New York Times*, "Although 120 of 138 medical schools say they are teaching communication skills, a great many of them do a very poor job."[4]

Lipkin believes, however, that effective interviewing is a skill that can be taught, one which amply rewards those who take the time to acquire it.

Lipkin's research indicates that in the most crucial moments of an interview—at the beginning and at the point where the patient is about to divulge what's really bothering him or her—the vast majority of doctors interrupt or dominate the conversation, cutting the patient off. Physicians typically do this *within the first eighteen seconds of the interview* as they follow a line of questioning ingrained during medical school training, based on the decision-tree method of determining a treatment plan. Typically, the patient's response is to stop giving information, reducing the doctor's ability to make a correct diagnosis.

While the doctor undoubtedly interrupts the patient in an attempt to obtain more precise information more quickly, his impatience may end up costing *more* time in making a diagnosis. At worst, the real underlying problem may never be divulged by a frustrated or frightened patient. The doctor familiar with effective interviewing techniques, on the other hand, is likely to gather the information needed to make a correct diagnosis, develop a better relationship with the patient, and keep costs down by eliminating unnecessary tests.

The effective medical interview elicits a full list of problems, an understanding of the patient's medical model of disease, and uncovers cultural beliefs that may stand in the way of compliance with treatment. The examination room exchange between doctor and patient also provides an opportunity to cement relationships with patients by setting a caring tone. The following are suggestions by various consultants and physicians for making the most of the medical interview.

Seeing Patients in Your Office

If you have been delayed or find that you are running late, apologize to patients when you get into the examining room. Let them know that you consider their time valuable.

Eliminate distraction and ensure privacy by turning off the television or radio, the phone, and the beeper, and by instructing staff to disturb you only for urgent problems.

Allow enough time in your schedule to fully explain procedures, diagnoses, medication instructions, the need for lab tests, and so on.

Always address patients by name. Ask them if they prefer to be addressed by their first name or surname. Begin the interview with "How are you feeling today, __________?"

Allow the patient to make his or her opening statement uninterrupted. Summarize what you've heard and then ask, "What else?" until the patient runs out of complaints. Often, the first complaint presented isn't the most important: get the whole story before developing hypotheses.

Organize the flow of the interview to elicit a narrative. Ask, "When did you last feel completely well?" or, "What happened as things changed with time?" You can interrupt to ask for more details, but then return to the narrative.

To survey the full range of problems, as well as the patient's feelings and beliefs about them, use such open-ended questions at the beginning of the interview as "Tell me more about that" or "How did that affect you?" If a patient complains of back pain, say, "Tell me about it," rather than asking closed-ended questions such as "Where?" or "Is it sharp or dull?"

Move from open-ended questions to closed-ended questions later in the interview. Closed-ended questions are the more focused questions such as "Did you smoke?" or "Is there heart disease in your family?" which require a yes, no, or other specific response.

Listen for barriers to compliance with treatment—for example, patients' medical and cultural beliefs.

Body language is also a form of communication. Fidgeting or looking at your watch says just as much as a smile or a reassuring gesture. This physical dimension of communication is an important variable in the medical interview. The most conducive position for interviewing a patient in the examining room, according to Lipkin, is for the doctor to sit with legs *un*crossed, in a relaxed position, making frequent, but not constant, eye contact with the patient.

Avoid medical jargon. No communication takes place unless there is an *exchange* of information. That means the patient must understand your explanations, your directions, and your prescription for treatment. Provide information in terms the patient can absorb.

Make sure the patient understands *why* he needs an upper GI series, *why* she must take the medication exactly three times a day, *why* she must take it with or without food. If possible, determine whether the treatment you prescribe fits with the patient's medical model (see below). If it does not, try to educate the patient, to change his or her medical model, or include some harmless element of the patient's model into the treatment plan, such as prescribing herbal tea or chicken soup in addition to your treatment plan.

Encourage patients to ask questions, and to discuss their health concerns and other matters—problems with your staff, your hours, whatever.

Compliment patients on their efforts to lose weight or

stop smoking, but don't criticize patients who are unable to do so.

Grant patients the dignity of being fully dressed when you discuss their problems and answer their questions.

Stay up to date on patients' family life and accomplishments. Clip articles from the local newspaper about your patients and place them in patient files, so you can comment on them at the next visit.

Allow 15-30 extra minutes for new patients. Introduce them to the staff, show them around the office, and have office policies and procedures explained to them.

Offer to make house calls for very sick or elderly patients who cannot come to see you.

Be generous with samples, especially if you are trying a new medication and want to see how the patient will tolerate it. If it's not the right medication for that patient, the sample will have saved the cost of a useless prescription and make your fee seem more reasonable.

Give patients both written and verbal guidelines on how to use the medications you prescribe. Help them to coordinate these with other medications they take.

Don't forget to ask if the patient has any questions.

Timing is important. Patients are most open to information at the beginning and end of a visit. Summarize what's been said and repeat your instructions at the end of the visit.

Take a moment to escort patients to the reception area or the door. Some office layouts can be confusing.

Seeing Hospitalized Patients

Many of the suggestions for office visits also apply to hospitalized patients. In addition, consider the following:

Doctors tend to spend more time at the nurses' station than in the patient's room. Reverse that order.

Spend at least fifteen minutes with your hospitalized patient on each visit, keeping in mind that you usually charge more for a hospital visit than for an office visit.

Sit at your patient's bedside rather than towering above a prone patient. The patient will perceive the visit to be longer than it actually is.

Don't hesitate to hold a frightened patient's hand.

Ask the patient if he or she has any questions, and offer explanations of procedures or tests ordered, treatment plans, and any other pertinent matters.

If one of your patients is hospitalized under the care of another physician, pay a courtesy call, without charge, to that patient. Explain that it isn't a professional call, but just a visit to see how he or she is getting along.

The Patient's Medical Model

Skilled interviewers discover and consider patients' own medical models, which influence patient feelings about their illness and its treatment. Failure to acknowledge the patient's health beliefs not only reduces the likelihood of cooperation with the prescribed treatment but also increases the risk of malpractice litigation later on. Lipkin, in an interview, gives the example of a Senegalese patient who presents with gastrointestinal complaints. The physician sends the patient off for an upper GI series, which comes back negative. The reason: Senegalese view their anatomy as consisting of one long tube and attribute their ailments to their "stomach," although the stomach may not be the source of their discomfort.

Or a patient comes in complaining of abdominal pain. When the interview begins, she emphasizes what she'd been eating when the pain began. The physician may want to ask about other possible causes of abdominal pain that have nothing to do with food. If he ignores the question of diet, however, the patient is likely to think the physician arrived at the wrong diagnosis.[5]

Dr. Michael Green takes herbs with him when he makes house calls. Working in a largely Hispanic area of New Mexico, where faith healers have been dispensing folk remedies for generations, Green knows that his ability to heal and his credibility with this population depend on his ability to bridge the gap between modern medicine and the old ways still practiced in his area. If he didn't respect local beliefs, chances are patients would not comply with the treatments he prescribes. A patient who does not comply—with potassium replacement therapy for his hypertension, for example—can get into serious trouble.

Who Has Control?

People from different cultural groups also have different expectations of the doctor-patient relationship. In Japan, patients expect to be told what to do by their doctors. Many recent immigrants, particularly those who view themselves as being in a lower class, also expect an authoritarian relationship, while American physicians often seek a partnership. For many cultures, the concept of a partnership is alien.

But even among American patients, a partnership concept may not succeed unless physicians guide patients in participating in their own care. Patients need to be taught what is going on with the disease and what is unknown, how they can influence its outcome, and how they can avoid limitations on their independence. Studies show that the majority of patients don't want to be involved in all the decisions about their care. The key is to sound patients out individually, to learn what role they want, and to realize that their wishes might change with time.[6]

Communication to Achieve Patient Satisfaction

In addition to anticipation of acknowledgment of their own health beliefs, patient expectations vary according to such elements of care as the amount of time spent by the doctor, amount of pain, waiting time, physician style, physician knowledge of family, and anticipation of future symptoms, among others.

Their satisfaction is linked to their perceptions of the physician and his or her practice, perceptions based on subjective opinions about such attributes as how friendly, caring, and competent a physician is. These opinions, in turn, are influenced by tangible evidence. Patients looking for a doctor they perceive to be competent will look at the physician's training, board certifications, honors received, hospital affiliations, offices held at the hospital and medical societies, and continuing education courses completed. Patients seeking an orthopedist who offers comprehensive service may look for the availablity of "wellness clinics" devoted to sports medicine within the practice.

In order to communicate so that patients are satisfied, then, physicians must get a sense of which of these factors people rely on in forming their opinions of the physician, and provide the corresponding tangible evidence. This can be accomplished informally at a first visit or through a patient brochure. Diplomas, certifications, and awards can be hung in a prominent location. Availability can be communicated by posting office hours, letting patients know how to reach the doctor after hours should an emergency arise, and making patients aware of coverage arrangements on weekends and vacations. Such tangible evidence lends credibility to any claim, stated or implied, made by the doctor, and ensures that patients' experiences will match their expectations. Promising to be available when needed, even if not in person, communicates more than just a fact: it communicates caring.

Although women are more likely than men to be satisfied with their physician, they change doctors more frequently, "shopping around" for a physician with whom they feel comfortable, studies conducted by the National Research Corporation show. Women are also more likely than men to have a chronic illness requiring medical care. Meeting women's expectations by effective communication can be an important consideration for many medical practices.

Coping with Patient Expectations

Patient satisfaction is also related to patient expectations of treatment outcome: getting results is a major factor in how satisfied patients are with a physician's competence, and getting good results is promoted through communication. Better results are reported when physician and patient are in agreement on diagnosis and treatment.

In discussing results, however, care must be taken not to raise patient expectations unrealistically, to avoid risking patient *dis*satisfaction with treatment outcome. Medical treatment often presents an ambiguous situation, making it difficult for the physician to impart with certainty and assurance what course the disease and treatment will take.

Under such circumstances, patients don't know whether to be satisfied or dissatisfied. The advice given by communication experts is that it is best to give patients understandable information about known aspects of the treatment.

Follow-up Communication

Even after an amicable doctor-patient visit, a patient may decide to transfer his or her health care to another physician, to disregard the physician's advice, or to skip or cancel the next appointment. Therefore, follow-up communication can be just as important in keeping patients in the practice as communication with them at the time of their visit (see chapter 4).

Call patients to relate results of lab tests (good and bad), to see how a patient is responding to treatment, and to consult with family members about a patient's condition. A personal phone call initiated by the doctor is one of the single most effective ways of making an impression on a patient. An after-visit phone call is a measure of special care. Because it is a relatively rare occurrence, it is something patients remember, a measure that cements good will. Consultants suggest that because so few physicians do it, after-visit phone calls to patients will lock in the patient base. Physicians who have made such calls find the positive response from patients to be a source of deep satisfaction.

But I Don't Have the Time

For many physicians, achieving a balance between economic forces and human relationships is difficult. An internist relates that he allows enough time in his schedule to talk with each patient, but his accountant tells him he should be seeing more patients each day. Relative to his peers, his income is down as a result of the way he practices.

In a more competitive environment, though, this

practice may prove to be rewarding. In a more competitive world, the edge will go to those providers who recognize the importance of knowing the patients as well as their diseases, says Robert Ebert, former dean of the Harvard Medical School.

Notes
1. *See* Ruffenach, p. 23. Reprinted by permission of the *Wall Street Journal*, © Dow Jones & Company, Inc. 1988. All Rights Reserved Worldwide.
2. Reprinted from *Health Care Management Review*, Vol. 13, No. 3, pp. 45-57, with permission of Aspen Publishers, Inc., © Summer 1988.
3. Lipkin, 1287.
4. Goleman, B1O.
5. Astrachan, 121.
6. *See* Lehman, 29.

6 DEVELOPING SOURCES OF REFERRALS

Referrals are a vital source of new patients for all physicians, and, barring any cataclysmic changes in reimbursement for health care delivery, they will undoubtedly continue to be a major basis for physician selection.

There are numerous ways in which people find providers of medical care. Many of the patients who consult a specialist are referred by their primary physician, while patients are likely to find general practitioners or pediatricians through a friend or relative. Some medical specialties, including ophthalmology, plastic surgery, and psychiatry, rely on self-referrals. Patients often find out about these services through publicity or advertising.

Personal referrals give patients much more confidence than such nonpersonal sources of information as advertising, Crane and Lynch found. A personal referral—from a friend, a relative, or another physician—so outweighed other important patient assessments of "competence," including the appearance of the office, that the latter may be entirely discounted by a consumer armed with a strong personal referral.

Referrals of new patients—whether from colleagues, from the practice's own patients, or from other sources in the community—can be increased. The tips that follow may help to keep your appointment book filled.

Increasing Referrals from Other Physicians

Socialize

Make efforts to meet more physicians in your community. Eat lunch at the local hospital cafeteria as often as possible—you may have to rearrange your schedule so that you are free around noon. Stop into the hospital's staff lounge or elsewhere in the hospital where physicians are likely to congregate, even for a couple of minutes, before returning to your office. Make yourself visible at hospital rounds, and attend hospital parties and functions.

Participate

Become active in organized medicine. Introduce yourself to colleagues at seminars, county medical society meetings, and continuing medical education courses. Join committees at your local hospital and attend their meetings.

Teach

Offer to conduct seminars, programs, and CME courses in your specialty or area of interest. Submit articles on these subjects to your county medical society newsletter or to state and specialty medical journals.

Write

Publish a quarterly newsletter on your specialty and send it to physicians who might refer patients to you. Include information on the latest developments in your specialty, such as new techniques and new drugs. Also include information about yourself and your staff.

Design a Brochure

Describe your specialty, scope of practice, affiliations, location, hours, payment policies, and anything else you consider important. Send it, along with a letter of welcome, to every new physician who comes to town. Also send it, along with a thank-you note, to any physician who refers a patient to you for the first time.

Accommodate

Reserve a few hours each week for new patients who have been referred by other physicians, so that you may see them quickly. Report back immediately to the referring physician, thank him or her for the referral, and keep that doctor apprised of the patient's progress. Take the time to write the physician a note for his or her file stating the diagnosis and treatment plan.

Return the Patient

Don't steal patients from a referring physician. Make a point of treating only those aspects of the patient's care for which he or she was referred to you—avoid repeating tests and procedures or attempting to treat other components of the patient's health. And don't criticize the care of the physician who referred the patient to you.

Refer to Others

Examine your own referral habits. Do you refer to younger practitioners because you assume established physicians are too busy? It's best not to make assumptions. Those who are too busy will ask you to refer the patient elsewhere, but will appreciate your thinking of them. To the extent possible, spread your referrals around evenly. If there are three gastroenterologists in town, refer patients to all three on a rotating basis—unless you have good reason not to refer to a particular person or group.

Have a Separate Phone Line

Consider having a private line just for physicians who want to discuss patients with you, so they are not kept waiting on busy office phones. If a separate line is not feasible, instruct your receptionist that calls from physicians are a priority: ask the person at the desk to put calls from doctors through to you if you are between office patients, or to page you if you are in the hospital, rather than take a message.

Make a practice of getting back to a physician who calls about a medical matter within as short a period of time as possible.

Provide Referral Forms

Make it easy for physicians to refer to you. One group of cardiologists supplies referring physicians with booklets containing twenty copies of forms (perforated for easy tearout) that require only that the referring physician's staff fill in the name and telephone number of the patient after calling the cardiologists to set up an appointment (see page 80). The front side of the forms gives the name and address of the cardiology group and directions to the office. The reverse side contains a description of the diagnostic test or procedure to be performed and instructions to the patient concerning the procedure. Different booklets are provided for stress tests, thallium stress tests, and echocardiograms.

Separate Diagnostic Lab from Your Office

If you are a specialist with a diagnostic lab that provides pulmonary function tests or stress tests—as opposed to routine blood work—consider treating the lab as a separate corporate entity and physically separating the lab from your office. A group of cardiologists found that referrals to their diagnostic lab increased dramatically after they moved the lab to a different location to allay referring physicians' fears that once a patient walks into a specialist's office, that patient will be lost.

Be Thoughtful

If you run across an article you think would be of interest to another physician, send him or her a copy.

Send Gifts

Sending holiday presents to referring physicians has

CARDIO DIAGNOSTICS OF FAIRFIELD

1305 Post Road, Suite 105
Fairfield, Connecticut 06430
(203) 255-9973

ECHOCARDIOGRAM

Patient's Name: ____________________

Date: ____________________________

Time: ____________________________

Referring Physician: _______________

DIRECTIONS:
I-95 to exit 22, turn south on North Benson Road. Go 2 short blocks to Post Road. Turn right on Post Road. Go about 1/4 mile to 3rd traffic light. Office entrance (Brickwalk) is located on the left diagonally across from the Post Office.

For Our Patient's Information:

An Echocardiogram is a sound wave picture of your heart. It allows us to easily obtain an accurate picture of the heart chambers, valves and muscle without radiation or side effects.

Because we will be examining the entire chest, please be sure to wear loose clothing.

FRONT ***BACK***

become commonplace. Fruit baskets, wine, or flowers show your appreciation for referrals sent throughout the year.

Increasing Referrals from Patients

Patient satisfaction is a key contributor to practice growth and stability. As one physician puts it, "Well-satisfied patients are the most effective means of practice building, and they cost me neither time nor money."[1]

For most fee-for-service physicians, word-of-mouth referrals from patients have been the primary means of promoting a practice's services. Studies show that two thirds of all new patients pick a physician on the recommendation of family and friends. The other third rely on various forms of advertising and promotion, including *Yellow Pages* listings, mailings, brochures, the sign outside the office, referral services, or referrals from colleagues.

Even when promotion is used, referrals from existing patients remain an important source of new patients. One medical group promoting their new walk-in clinic with a "media miniblitz" found that referrals from existing patients were the second largest source of new patients, right behind a direct-mail campaign conducted by a public relations expert.

Consultants suggest the following to increase referrals from current patients.

Track Referrals

Ask new patients to indicate on their information sheet how they found out about you. This will give you a good idea of your best referral sources, and might suggest other sources to cultivate. If your patients are not high among your referral sources, consider a consultation with a communication specialist.

Thank Patients

Send a note or call to thank patients who refer other patients to your practice.

Send Gifts

Some patients refer numerous friends, neighbors, and relatives to a practice. A gift certificate to a local restaurant, flowers, a plant, a fruit basket, a magazine subscription, conveys your appreciation for their unsolicited promotion of your practice.

Distribute Brochures

Keep a good supply of patient information brochures in the reception area. Patients often take home brochures describing the practice, the specialty or specific procedures performed to show or give to friends and relatives.

Cultivate Non-Physician Providers

Many practices find that a significant number of referrals come from podiatrists, nurses, chiropractors, and pharmacists.

Send thank-you notes for their referrals.

If you have a newsletter, add their names to your mailing list.

Consider developing an in-service training course for nurses and others who require credits toward relicensure.

Refer patients to them.

Notes

1. Erhardt, 81.

7 PREPARING PATIENT EDUCATION MATERIALS

Many physicians are aware they are not the primary source of health care information for their patients. Rather than turning to their doctors for information on health-related matters, patients rely on newspapers, magazines, television, and friends for health information and for clarification of health care issues in the news.

Because patients are now more interested in health matters, many doctors have decided to play a larger role in providing health information to their patients and community, in helping patients to prevent diseases and motivating patients to take responsibility for their health. Some physicians have decided to speak out on the broader issues of delivery of health care, its costs, its capabilities and limitations.

Providing such information often involves production of written and audiovisual materials, so many physicians need and seek outside assistance. Of five hundred physicians surveyed by the National Research Corporation, 40 percent said they would increase admissions to hospitals that provided them with assistance in preparing tools for health education. Physicians cited brochures, videotapes, health newsletters, and other communication services aimed at patients as the type of materials they most needed help preparing.

Patient education and health promotion materials typically serve four primary purposes:

- Increase patient and community knowledge about the practice.
- Increase patient, community, and colleagues' knowledge of the medical specialty.
- Increase patient and community knowledge of health matters.
- Create a supportive climate for private medical practice.

What to Communicate: The Big Picture

The medical profession must convince Democrats to avoid national health insurance, and Republicans that DRGs are not a competitive system, according to Walter McClure, president of the Center for Policy Studies. Unless they can do so successfully, McClure told doctors, "either 100 percent of you will take a 20 percent loss in income, which I doubt, or 80 percent of you will push the other 20 percent over the edge."[1]

Whether the arena is the legislature, the media, the public at large, or the doctor-patient relationship, the ultimate goal of communication efforts is to create a climate of support for fee-for-service physicians. Physicians want to have a more balanced view of medicine presented—its true costs, its demand on the physician's time, and its responsibilities, both legal and moral, "neither overlooking its deficiencies, overpromising its accomplishments, nor making it appear inept and self-serving."[2]

They want people to know how government regulations make it expensive and clumsy to practice medicine. And they want patients and others to know why their doctors can provide better, more economical care than is possible under any national health insurance program.

Quality of health care is another important and little understood health care issue. Quality health care, McClure said, has little to do with cost. In some cases quality, if defined as doing more and spending more on a patient, may even decline, as when undergoing a procedure puts a patient at risk of such dangerous side effects as nosocomial infections.

The key message, which serves as the stated theme of many medical associations, is that if quality is to remain high, delivery of medical care is best left in the hands of qualified physicians.

What Americans Want to Learn

Americans have their own notions of what they want to hear about from physicians. An AMA poll found that 93 percent of the public named child abuse as an important issue for physicians to address. Other issues they rated as very important were the marketing of alcoholic beverages (77%), environmental health hazards (67%), patients' rights to refuse treatment (66%), and the effects of television and movie violence on children (55%).

The concerns of special interest groups present another opportunity for physicians to state their views on medical issues. Among the most powerful of these groups is the nation's elderly, who lobby for more home care, better ambulatory care, and for medical care to be provided in continuing care communities.

What the Media and Doctors Want to Convey

The content of the messages doctors ought to communicate has been the subject of lively discussion by the media and by physicians, as the following quotes illustrate:

> There are continuing battles to be fought. But physicians should pick their ground carefully. There are reforms that would make the health system more efficient, more responsive, more economical. I think it is important for the medical profession to show a willingness to accept such changes.
>
> —*Newspaper editor John Grace*

> We must offer tangible evidence to our patients that there will be a doctor available, and we will relieve their pain and suffering, and that we will do our best, without compromise.
>
> —*Vernon Astler, M.D.*
> *past president, Florida Medical Association*

> Pesticides, drug abuse, pollutants, et cetera, are creating serious problems and a menace to health . . . . Many physicians just have not had time or have not taken time to exert their influence in the community in matters of public health that are of serious concern to us all.
>
> —*Henry Bockus, M.D.*
> *delivering a distinguished lecture*

> Doctors must learn that it is honorable to speak out to the press, to provide facts, to correct errors,

> and to give reasonable testimony on controversial issues. Stop looking at those who do it honorably as publicity seekers . . . . As long as the responsible leaders keep silent, the quacks and charlatans will fill the vacuum.
>
> —*Lawrence Altman*
> *physician and full-time*
> New York Times *medical reporter*

What to Communicate About Your Practice

Physicians just getting their feet wet in the patient education or marketing world frequently have trouble deciding what information to communicate about themselves. Many don't see the necessity of highlighting characteristics that they themselves have long since taken for granted.

Most consultants agree that when considering alternative messages to use in brochures and newsletters, the less aggressive approach is usually preferable. Factual, objective, tangible information about the practice is more acceptable, more credible, and more effective than making claims about competence (quality of care) or caring. Basic information, such as services available, location, and office hours takes precedence over everything else. However, secondary information, which can often be the deciding factor in bringing in business, should be included.

In any communication effort, doctors should convey in an honest, straightforward fashion, the following aspects of their practices, according to consultants Glenys Piesto and Wayne Redding:

Anything New

This includes new personnel, new equipment, new services, new billing procedures, and new office decor.

Anything Special

Unique services your practice offers should be communicated. Some examples include nontraditional office hours—a real benefit to many current and potential patients—or free classes, such as evening parenting classes and free Saturday morning joggers' clinics, which can attract new patients and increase the perception of value among the patients you see.

Personal Attributes

Does your office project ultraprofessionalism? Refreshing efficiency? A personal, caring attitude? Technological savvy? You may not be unique in your specialty, but you are unique in other ways. Let people know your special qualities.

Your Philosophy of Medicine

Do you subscribe to a particular school of thought? Do you have a holistic approach? Do you have attitudes toward your specialty, or the practice of medicine, that you enjoy sharing with friends and colleagues? Be careful in the way you communicate them to the public, but by all means do so.

Medical Developments

You keep abreast of developments in your field, and the public generally does not. You will be doing a public service, and a service to your practice, by disseminating noteworthy information about medical research and progress.

Conservative Communication Vehicles

Brochures

Brochures have many uses: they can describe your practice, provide health care information, or deliver a message—for example, why it is important to see your regular doctor who knows you rather than the stranger you are apt to encounter in a walk-in center.

Brochures should be as brief as possible and written on the level of the intended reader. Because they can be expensive to produce, before you start you should:

- Identify the specific purpose of each brochure.

- Think about the distribution method.

- Specify the intended audience.

A brochure describing your practice can be anything from a neatly typed sheet for a small practice to a full-color brochure for a large group practice.

The most practical size is one that fits nicely into a business-size envelope. Typically, a brochure consists of an 8 1/2" x 11" sheet of paper folded in thirds. If it is to be mailed without an envelope, one panel has to be available for the address. This panel usually includes a preprinted return address and the bulk mail indicia.

A practice brochure (see pages 90–91) should contain the following information:

- A description of the full range of services

- An explanation of your specialty

- Office hours; times set aside for certain types of visits

- Policy on cancellations, late appointments, callbacks

- Location (with a map if necessary)

- Whom to call for appointments, for non-emergency

Sally O'Brien, M. D.

Dr. O'Brien received her medical degree from Stanford University following undergraduate studies at the University of Massachusetts, Amherst. She completed her residency in internal medicine at Tufts–New England Medical Center and is board certified in internal medicine. Before moving to Hollywood, she served as assistant professor of medicine at Tufts University Medical School. She is a member of the L. A. County Medical Society and the American College of Physicians.

Nathan E. Goldberg, M. D.

Dr. Goldberg received his undergraduate degree from the Massachusetts Institute of Technology and his medical degree from the University of Pennsylvania. He completed his residency in internal medicine at the Medical College of Virginia and is board certified in internal medicine. Before settling in Hollywood, he practiced two years in LaPlace, Louisiana, for the National Health Service Corps. He is a member of the L. A. County Medical Society and the American College of Physicians.

Sally O'Brien, M. D.
Nathan E. Goldberg, M. D.
Hollywood Medical Center
1462 Vine St.
Hollywood, CA 90028

Medical Office of
Sally O'Brien, M. D.
461-9355
and
Nathan E. Goldberg, M. D.
461-6100

Hollywood Medical Center
1462 Vine St.
Hollywood, CA 90028

Sample Brochure: Outside

Sample Brochure: Inside

Welcome to Our Medical Office
This brochure contains information about our practice—who we are, what kind of medical problems we treat, how to contact us, and many other details. If you have any comments or questions, please let us know. We would be happy to talk with you.

What Sort of Medical Problems Do We Treat?
We are both board certified in internal medicine, and we treat the full range of adult medical problems. As generalists, we are concerned about the whole person. We provide you with comprehensive health care and a personalized approach to problems that require the services of specialists.

How to Reach the Doctors
When you call our office, our trained assistant will discuss your medical problems with you and relay your message to your doctor. Please be sure to provide our assistant with complete information so that we can help you quickly and appropriately. To help us respond promptly, our nurse will often be the first one to return your call.

On nights and weekends, we share coverage with Dr. Richard Howards and Dr. Scott Andrews, both of Los Angeles. One of us will always be available to return your call. Simply call our office (either number). The phone is answered 24 hours a day.

Emergencies and Urgent Problems
There is always a doctor from our coverage group available to answer your questions or meet you at our office, his office, the medical walk-in center or the hospital emergency room. In case of emergency, you need not wait to reach one of us by telephone Call for an ambulance or go directly to the Hollywood Presbyterian Medical Center Hospital Emergency Room. Once there, tell them that we are your doctors, and they will notify us.

Scheduling Appointments
Our trained assistant will talk with you to find out what type of appointment you need. Certain types of appointments, such as yearly physicals, will be scheduled well in advance.

For urgent or episodic problems such as "the flu," we will fit you into our schedule, usually the same day. Please describe the nature of your problem to our assistants so that we can schedule you for the appropriate time with the doctor. We are usually "on time" for office visits, so it is helpful if you can arrive a few minutes before your appointment. If you cannot keep an appointment, please call us as soon as you know, even if it is the same day or the same hour as the appointment. If our schedule is disrupted by emergencies, we will make every effort to contact you.

Prescriptions
Prescriptions will be written with sufficient refills to last you through your next scheduled office visit. If a prescription should run low, please call your pharmacy before it runs out to see if they have refill instructions in their records. If the pharmacy is unable to refill your prescription, please call us during office hours so that we will have access to your medical record.

Hospital
We are both on staff and have admitting privileges at Hollywood Presbyterian Medical Center and Beverly Palms Rehabilitation Hospital.

Nursing Home Care
We care for nursing home patients in the Los Angeles area.

House Calls
In general, we can serve you best in our office where we have access to the equipment and tests often required for accurate diagnosis and treatment. However, we do make house calls in Hollywood when it is appropriate (for example, home-bound patients).

Payment
Payment is expected at the time of your office visit. Our fee schedule is available upon request. We accept cash and personal checks. There is a $10 charge for returned checks. If you have a problem paying a bill within 30 days, please discuss this with our office manager. She can arrange an extended payment schedule for you.

Medicare, Major Health Plans
We both participate in Medicare and all major health plans. You are responsible for the fraction of our fee that your plan expects you to pay. Details for each plan are complex and change frequently. Specific information for patients with Medicare will be provided to you by our staff.

Blue Cross/Blue Shield and Commercial Health Insurance
Patients with Blue Cross/Blue Shield or commercial health insurance are expected to pay for office visits at the time services are rendered. At the end of each monthly billing period, if you request it, we will provide you with receipts to submit to your insurance company for reimbursement. Detailed information about insurance reimbursement for office and hospital services will be provided to you by our staff.

Preventive Medicine and Good Health
We have a special interest in helping you to maximize your overall health and fitness. This can be achieved through attention to diet, exercise, health habits, and appropriate use of screening tests. We will work with you to develop an individualized plan to help you reach your health and fitness goals.

clinical advice, for prescription refills, and for test results

- How to reach you after hours

- Your coverage arrangements, when absent

- Billing policies and procedures

- A paragraph or two about each provider, listing credentials and, if desired, philosophy

To maximize the reach and effectiveness of both practice and health education brochures, follow these suggestions:

Imprint or stamp the physician or group name on the cover of all health education brochures and pamphlets that are not produced by or specifically for the practice.

Where needed, provide translated material in the appropriate language(s).

In a patient education brochure, cover topics pertinent to the medical problems you see in your practice and to disease prevention and wellness.

Many brochures are available at little or no cost from the American Heart Association, American Lung Association, and similar organizations.

The American Heart Association, for example, provides a catalogue listing all its available brochures, including its popular diet. These brochures are available to physicians at cost ($5.18 per 100 brochures).

Newsletters

A newsletter can be a valuable investment for a physician. It serves two purposes: to inform its audience of the services provided by the physician and to provide valuable public education to patients. Newsletters should come across as informational rather than promotional.

A newsletter may project a "high-tech" or a "high-touch" image—or any position in between. No matter what the approach, the tone of the newsletter should fit the practice.

To be successful, a newsletter directed to patients must contain timely information of interest to the people reading it. The lead article, the most newsworthy item in the issue, should appear on the front page. The newsletter may also feature excerpts from medical journals, news of staff members' families, or Mrs. Cohen's recipe for chicken soup. Articles should be short, and the average reader should be able to understand every word. If a newsletter is geared to patients, appearance is usually as important as content, consultants advise. At the very least, it should look professional.

Those practices concerned with image development should consider seeking professional advice on producing materials for public distribution. For the do-it-yourself practice equipped with a computer, many inexpensive software programs are available to help you produce a reasonable newsletter.

Do-it-yourselfers might also benefit from Tom Lichty's *Design Principles for Desktop Publishing* (Scott Foresman & Co., $19.95), which introduces basic design principles, teaches readers how to produce attractive, well-designed publications, and offers many humorous examples.

A number of companies provide generic newsletters containing professionally written articles with your practice name on the masthead. Though this type of newsletter looks professional, it may be too generic. The articles may not reflect your medical and practice philosophy or give you the option of including newsworthy items about your own practice.

Distribution

Generally, newsletters are sent to current patients. They may be distributed along with the monthly bills to help reduce mailing costs, in which case they should be sized to fit billing envelopes. If you would like to increase readership of your practice's newsletter, the following suggestions may be useful:

- Publicize free subscriptions with fliers placed at local hospitals, pharmacies, community centers, and other public places.
- Place an ad in your local paper indicating the newsletter is available.
- Collect names and addresses of persons who might be interested in your newsletter; for example, people who attend a talk by a member of your practice could provide the beginning of such a mailing list.

Newsletters for Colleagues

Some physicians find it useful to write a quarterly newsletter for other physicians. Send the newsletter to colleagues who are likely to refer patients, and include information on the latest developments in your specialty. New techniques, new drugs, and new technology are among the many possible topics. Include information about yourself and your staff to let other physicians know what your practice has to offer.

Bill Stuffers

A simpler alternative to a newsletter is to include notes with monthly bills. Use these to let patients know about new staff, changes in office hours, any awards/citations/courses completed by practice personnel, or anything you think might be of interest to your patients. Make copies of bill stuffers available in the waiting and examining rooms for patients who pay at the time of the visit and do not receive bills.

Slide Presentations

Skip the slides of the family trip to China. If, however, you traveled to China to learn a new technique related to your specialty, set aside a few evenings and invite patients to the office for a slide presentation to show them how the new technique can be beneficial to them. Consider a session or two for referring physicians as well, again stressing patient benefits.

Videotapes

With videocassette recorders commonplace in American homes, VCR tapes provide an opportunity for patients to take the doctor home with them. Tapes made specifically for the practice are a particularly advantageous approach for practices wishing to portray a "high-tech" image.

In this age of "how-to" videotapes, consider preparing a videotape lending library. Topics should be relevant to your practice and informative to patients. Give first consideration to recommended treatments and techniques patients often have difficulty understanding or adhering to.

Some topics particularly suited to visual media include how-tos for identifying abnormal reactions to medication, treatment instructions, and diagnostic checks, such as breast self-examination. A pulmonary physician might inform patients on the proper use and care of nebulizers and inhalers, while an obstetrician might prepare a tape outlining the pregnancy, labor, and delivery process. Patients shown exercises for an injured knee at a morning appointment might not remember the precise instructions by evening. Did he say sit up or lie down to do this exercise? Am I supposed to hold my leg in that position for a while or keep moving it up and down? Is that the rash she told me to watch out for or is this just dry skin? A tape could answer such questions and perhaps cut down on the number of calls to your office.

If you give a talk in the community, consider having the presentation taped and made available to interested patients who are unable to attend the lecture.

Look under "Video Production Services" in the *Yellow Pages* directory for firms that produce videos. If you are making a video for your patients' home use, be sure to specify half-inch tape: most professionals use three-quarter-inch tapes that cannot be viewed on home VCR equipment.

Recorded video presentations on a variety of general health topics, such as exercise and nutrition, are available for loan from medical libraries and from medical organizations. You can also contact companies that lend or sell films, or you can tell your patients about them.

General Considerations

Like audiovisual materials, written materials can be either custom produced or simply purchased from medical associations and drug companies. Some physicians prepare such materials themselves, sometimes with the assistance of graphic arts and communication students from local colleges. Others hire hospital public relations staff members—on a freelance basis—or professional firms to prepare materials for the practice.

Always remember the target audience when you review brochures, newsletters, videotapes, or other patient education materials. A newsletter to referring physicians is usually written on a different level from one slated for distribution to patients.

Keep in mind when preparing such materials that women are far more likely than men to select a physician when illness occurs in a family, when surgery is required by a family member, and when a physician is chosen for their own and their children's health care. On the other hand, men are more likely than women to choose a provider for treatment of injuries to adults and for their own illnesses.

Printing costs for brochures, newsletters, pamphlets, and other printed patient education materials vary widely. It pays to get bids from several printers.

A do-it-yourself approach saves typesetting charges, which can be considerable. Notices and other patient education materials can be produced in-house with an ordinary typewriter and either a lettering machine (available from most office supply companies) or rub-off transfer letters, such as Letraset.

Some practices develop a logo for all their printed materials: business cards, envelopes, letterhead stationery, prescription pads, memo pads. Logos are used to aid recognition of the practice and to portray an image.

If you decide to use a logo, make sure it portrays the image you want to cultivate.

Distributing Patient Education Materials

In the Office

Keep practice brochures and patient education materials in the waiting room. Buy a special holder, available through medical office supply catalogues, for a neat display.

Specific instructional material may be handed to appropriate patients by the doctor or other staff member.

Outside the Office

Mail your practice brochure to new patients when

John S. Grant, M.D.
123 Main Street
Anytown, U.S.A.

Dear Mr. Patient:

Welcome to our practice. We appreciate the opportunity to serve you.

We are enclosing a copy of our patient information handbook. Please take the time to look it over. It contains information about our practice that will help you use our services to your full advantage. If you have any questions, please give us a call; Dr. Grant will be happy to speak to you.

You will find that we can assist you in many ways regarding your health. We can help you find other medical specialists if you need them, include you in our ongoing educational programs, and share with you general information about maintaining good health. Please don't hesitate to let us know how we can best serve you.

Sincerely,

John S. Grant, M.D., and Staff

they make an appointment, along with your "welcome" letter (see sample above) and a confirmation of the appointment.

Newsletters, as previously mentioned, may be more widely distributed to interested persons throughout the community.

Brochures or newsletters can also be mailed to the following audiences, often identified in the research phase preceding a communication plan:

- Industry
- Civic groups
- Other physicians in the community who might refer patients
- Area housing developments (for the elderly, for young families, and those that attract yuppies)
- Chamber of Commerce and other local business groups
- Charitable organizations
- Religious institutions and facilities
- Boy Scouts, Girl Scouts, and other youth groups
- Welcome Wagon
- Realtors
- Schools
- Health and human service organizations in the community
- Hotels and motels

Direct mail is a subtle, personalized, and economical way to communicate a message. Use it for practice brochures or other communication. Direct mail is used most frequently to attract new patients to a practice, and mass mailing may be a useful technique for new physicians, or those with new images or information to convey. One of the major advantages of direct mail is that it enables the physician to target specific audiences.

For example, an obstetrician/gynecologist may mail a letter or brochure to all new female residents of selected neighborhoods in the service area. Another advantage is that the effectiveness of a direct-mail campaign is easily measured—simply ask new patients how they were referred to the practice, and keep a tally of those who came in as a result of mail received.

Mailing lists for a direct-mail campaign can be developed or purchased for particular zip codes, age groups, income groups, and so on. One medical practice had a direct mail firm send a brochure to every household within two miles of the practice. Firms that specialize in direct mail are listed in the *Yellow Pages* under "Advertising—Direct Mail." Such firms offer a range of services, including design, production, printing, addressing, sorting, and even bundling mailings into zip codes to take advantage of reduced mailing rates, which are available for a mailing of five hundred or more letters (a mailing permit is required).

Notes
1. *See* L. Page, 14.
2. I.H. Page, 645.

8 COMMUNITY SERVICE

For physicians seeking to build or consolidate their practices, high public visibility is an important means to this end. Properly approached, it may also prove invaluable to the medical profession's reputation. An image of community participation and social responsibility may be just the shot in the arm the medical profession needs at a time when the future of medical practice is being publicly weighed.

"We as doctors have lost some of our magic . . . things have really changed. We're being sued. What does that mean? It means that people don't trust us. We're being castigated as a group for making too much money and not caring enough," said Dr. Thomas Delbanco of Boston's Beth Israel Hospital on the public television program *NOVA*.

Though doctors—and the American medical establishment as it is presently constituted—have their admirers, it is not the fans who are shouting the loudest. Rather, it is those who are disgruntled with some aspect of medical care, be it quality or cost.

Physicians, too, are caught in soul-searching. They are often quite hard on themselves. Receiving a meritorious service award from the American College of Emergency Physicians, Dr. Jack Page of Charleston, West Virginia, used the occasion to berate physicians for their income gains. As doctors' compensation increases, he told his colleagues, society's respect for them decreases. American physicians are losing sight of their purpose for existence, and, having lost their sense of social responsibility, are becoming nothing more than skilled tradesmen, like plumbers or electricians, he added. As a result, society perceives American physicians as self-serving and self-centered, perceptions that have had significant negative impact on the profession.

Physicians have good reason *not* to participate in the affairs of their communities. Some may lack the skills needed to communicate effectively in a public forum. But for most, the problem is a need for more cost-effective use of time and resources, a force that dictates against time spent communicating. Pulled in three different directions by their professional duties to patients, their families, and their communities, physicians resent their civic duties most. They feel that they make their contributions to the community through their profession rather than through other good works. In addition, says Robert Ebert, their medical school training, for the most part, teaches values that involve one-to-one relationships with patients rather than dealing with broader health care issues. In any case, the reluctance of physicians to devote time to promoting patient and community understanding of their views on major medical issues and to show their sense of social responsibility more publicly may be at the heart of the public perception that physicians are more devoted to the business side of their practices than to patient care.

According to Lamar Soutter, former dean of the University of Massachusetts Medical School, the deterioration of the physician's image in the public eye in the past twenty years is a result of the fact that, collectively, physicians are regarded as rich, self-interested, and indifferent to public need. His prescription for a new image: concerned participation in community affairs. If doctors continue to be viewed merely as purveyors of expensive services, he said, they will be unable to forestall the advent of national health insurance and further legislative restrictions on the practice of medicine. Constraints placed on physicians depend as much on how great an interest they have shown in society as on how well they have served as doctors, he argued.

"We physicians are not terribly involved in our communities, which is a shame, because we have a lot to offer," echoes Josef Fischer, chairman of the Department of Surgery at the University of Cincinnati Medical Center and a graduate of Harvard Medical School.

Patient education is known to save on overall health care costs, increase patient compliance with treatment, and improve the physician-patient relationship. Patient education activities, though they may require a commitment of time, can be of enormous benefit to the physician's practice, as well as to the reputation of the medical profession.

Community Involvement

Involvement must have as its primary purpose the improvement of health in the physician's community. Community service for physicians means public speaking engagements for the purpose of educating the community about health-related issues. It means participation in free health screenings and health fairs. It may involve providing funds to community causes and joining community organizations.

Those physicians who are highly visible in their communities often make major gains in attracting new patients to their practices. But even for the thriving practice, community involvement has benefits. It not only helps maintain the patient base but also enhances the reputation and image of the physician.

For physicians with full practices, these benefits may not become evident until a future time. But when and if competition in the practice area heats up, it is they who will have that all-important edge. Having one's name before the public in a positive light can be regarded as an insurance policy as third-party payers continue to tighten their belts.

There are many ways, some requiring more time than others, to become involved in community affairs. Communication professionals suggest the following:

Volunteer. Sit on boards and committees of local organizations—the board of education, community centers, groups providing food and shelter for the homeless. Choose organizations and committees for whom your medical expertise or your contacts can be a valuable asset. For example, fund-raising organizations, such as the United Way, have found that when physicians call other physicians for donations, they obtain better results. And many of the schools and community organizations that are now scrambling to create AIDS policies could use the medical input of a practicing physician.

Join. Being part of civic and community groups will help you become an active and well-known member of your local community. If you reside some distance from the community in which you work, make your presence felt in your work community. Join the local Chamber of Commerce or other groups. Involvement is the traditional way for physicians to get their names out, and it is still among the most successful practice builders for new or flagging practices.

Speak. Join your local medical society's or hospital's speakers bureau. Make presentations to civic groups, parents' clubs, senior citizens groups, business groups, and religious organizations, on timely topics related to your specialty, if those groups contain potential patients for your practice. Though these speaking engagements are usually coordinated most successfully through speakers bureaus, you can also offer to speak to condominium groups and neighborhood and community associations. Speaking opportunities include formal speeches, luncheon talks, guest lectures, panel discussions, and question-and-answer sessions.

Write. Write a newspaper column about health issues or about your specialty (see chapter 12, "Getting Media Attention").

Participate in Health Fairs. Provide free cataract, blood pressure, pulmonary function screenings or other services when your local hospital sponsors a health fair.

Undertake Community Service Projects. Help with school health or immunization programs and community health screenings. Volunteer to be a team physician, to coach a neighborhood soccer or baseball team, or to be a consultant to local schools or nursing homes. Sponsor local sports teams or school scholarships.

Educate. Participate in or sponsor community health education courses—for instance, in CPR, first aid, seasonal allergies.

Engage in Politics. Consider running for elected office, or volunteer to serve on a community health board or other commission that interests you.

More about Speaking Engagements

Physicians who can speak effectively without using medical jargon and who enjoy educating people are those who find speaking engagements an enjoyable as well as profitable investment of time. The key is to speak primarily to audiences you wish to attract to your practice. Once you have established your "target market," the local Chamber of Commerce can provide you with a list of women's, professional, fraternal, and business organizations.

State and local government agencies are another source of information about organized groups in your practice area. If your target market is, for example, the elderly, local agencies serving this population can lead you to groups and clubs for senior citizens.

Speakers bureaus vary in effectiveness. John Ferretti, an Erie, Pennsylvania, internist, reported that after he signed up with a local speakers bureau, months went by without his receiving a single request to speak. A speakers bureau organized by the public relations department of your local hospital or a public relations consultant serving the health care field may be a better resource.

Whenever you speak to a group, be sure to have attendees sign in. Ask for names and addresses. Add these to your mailing list, to be used for announcing new services, new offices, or sending a newsletter.

Part III

A MORE AGGRESSIVE COMMUNICATION STRATEGY

In pursuing patient education activities, some physicians may do no more than develop practice brochures that provide handy office information for current patients. Yet the patient education and health promotion activities discussed in the previous section provide an opportunity to go a step further, beyond the office into the community, in a more organized effort to attract new patients to a practice. A more aggressive communication strategy maintains the focus on patients and on education, but searches for more "bang for the buck."

Part III defines those communication activities suitable for the medical practice that wants to attract patients and referrals without resorting to advertising.

9 COMPETITION: AN IMPETUS TO STEP UP MARKETING

According to AMA figures, there are approximately half a million physicians in the United States today, double the number of the 1950s. That number increases each year by the addition of seventeen thousand new M.D.s trained in U.S. institutions and over three thousand trained abroad. The number of doctors per ten thousand people increased from fourteen in 1960 to nineteen in 1980, a ratio predicted to grow to twenty-five physicians per ten thousand people by 1990. Despite the growing number of physicians who retire early or change careers, the ranks of physicians are swelling. By the year 2000 a surplus of physicians is likely, the Institute for the Future predicts. To some, these numbers point to a physician glut, a matter of concern to many physicians.

Pros and Cons of Physician Surplus

Not all physicians view their increasing numbers as a threat. One advantage is improved quality of care, says John Sandson, former dean of Boston University Medical School. On the positive side, he cites an increase in primary care physicians, more physicians moving to previously underserved areas, and a greater number of minority physicians entering practice.

But for many physicians, the trend spells competition. More than half the Pennsylvania physicians surveyed in a recent study expect competitive pressures to increase.[1] Nationwide, more and more physicians tell the AMA that they are concerned about competition, and that economic competition is too high.

For those just starting out in practice, competition means that much greater effort must be expended to get the phone to ring. It means that they may not be able to locate the new practice according to their personal preference, as physicians did in the past. Today, selecting a location must be more carefully considered, taking into account whether the physician will be able to survive in a chosen area. "The time is rapidly approaching," Sandson predicted, "when the demand for some specialists at hospitals in major urban areas will be exhausted, while others will find it nearly impossible to establish practices in many cities across the country."

Even established physicians can no longer count on keeping their current patient population intact without taking steps to ensure patient satisfaction. An AMA poll found that mid-career physicians felt particularly threatened by competition: 49 percent of physicians forty-five to fifty-four years old rated competition as "too high."

This is not surprising, considering that sources of competition have increased vastly in recent years. An obstetric practice now competes with midwives, birth centers, and at-home deliveries supervised by nurse-practitioners. Physicians in private practice are surrounded by HMOs, surgical centers, and walk-in clinics. According to the AMA, declining practices are on the rise in large cities (population 5 million or more), with general practitioners hardest hit. Female physicians, however, are more likely to report an increasing patient load than their male counterparts.

Competition from Alternative Health Care Providers

As yet, with the exception of some specialities in some cities, competition has not become intense among physicians in private practice. But as the number of practicing doctors continues to increase, it almost certainly will. "This will have an impact on referrals to specialists and on the ability of the solo practitioners, or even small, single-specialty group practice, to survive," said Robert Ebert, now special adviser to the president of the Robert Wood Johnson Foundation, an organization whose purpose is to improve health services in the United States.

Of greater immediate concern to physicians is competition from the growth of such alternatives to traditional fee-for-service physician services as HMOs, independent practice associations, surgical and trauma centers, and hospital outpatient services and satellite clinics. Sophisticated management, aggressive marketing, and greater flexibility in tailoring care to the special needs of patients give these corporate health care providers certain advantages. With competition of this type, and with non-M.D. practitioners also luring patients away, physicians often need the help of professionals to maintain their patient base.

Marketing in the Face of Competition

The economic laws of supply and demand apply to medicine as they do to other economic activity, according to economist Rita Ricardo-Campbell of the Hoover Institution. Although this may seem self-evident to economists and to the business community, it is a new concept for many physicians.

"Competition is more than a new word for us. It is an altered way of life," William Kissick, professor of public health at the University of Pennsylvania, told a meeting of physicians, medical scientists, and corporate executives. Competition, he added, is a product of the change in health care from a social good to a market good.

Physicians are beginning to absorb the new reality and are making an effort to respond to it. More and more, office-based doctors are responding by launching marketing efforts.

Albuquerque, New Mexico, internist Alan Zelicoff told the *Wall Street Journal* that he and his colleagues find themselves spending several hours a week discussing such things as marketing strategies and new income sources. They do not relish this added burden. "Not only am I uninterested in this task, I am completely unprepared for it," he said. "Yet if we aren't aggressive in the marketplace, we will be unable to practice the skills we spent eight years perfecting."[2]

Where competition is keen, patient recruitment, marketing, public relations, and promotion are words that are quickly creeping into physicians' vocabularies. A growing number of doctors, many of them young and in the process of establishing practices, are finding that it's no longer sufficient to hang out a shingle and expect patients to come flocking into the waiting room. Instead, young doctors find that they have to market their practices to attract—and keep—patients, and that patient loyalty has to be earned.

Young physicians entering private practice, faced with debts and with the soaring cost of malpractice insurance, are especially in need of practice recruitment strategies.

By 1990, as the number of patients per doctor is expected to fall to 30 percent below 1975 levels, the gains of any one physician will increasingly come at the expense of another, in what Paul Starr, author of *The Social Transformation of American Medicine*, calls a zero-sum game. Consequently, many physicians are proving not at all reluctant to pay professionals hefty fees to help them design and implement patient strategies. As far back as 1983, the *Wall Street Journal* was reporting that physicians in Los Angeles, Manhattan, and other towns in New York were paying public relations agencies from $1,500 to $2,500 a month to publicize their practices and arrange television and radio appearances.[3]

"For most doctors, marketing is a dirty word," says David Zeitlin, an executive of the Los Angeles County Medical Association. "I think the average doctor thinks, 'I'm not a marketer. I'm not a huckster. I'm a doctor.' He's not being realistic."[4]

Physician Discomfort with Marketing

Even when they seek professional counsel, physicians frequently attempt to dissociate themselves from marketing efforts. Medicine is supposed to be above such things, most doctors feel. But despite the pervasive opinion that advertising and other promotional tools are ill suited to the medical profession's image, competition often forces physicians' hands. "I've had doctors tell me they want public relations, but don't tell anybody my name," said Susan Tellem, president of Los Angeles-based Grody/Tellem Communications, a medical marketing firm.[5]

"There's a feeling of wanting to do something, but on the other hand a fear of what their peers will say about it," Tellem said. Indeed, a urologist who employed a public relations agency told the *Wall Street Journal* that he kept it a secret, fearing loss of referrals from other physicians.[6] Tellem believes that medicine is a business and should avail itself of common business strategies. She believes all doctors need at least a marketing plan, advice echoed by many consultants.

But some doctors find this advice hard to swallow. Surveys have found that a large majority of them believe, quite contrary to the marketing literature, that marketing is a synonym for advertising. Because advertising evokes strong negative sentiments, this dislike is unnecessarily extended to marketing in general. Advertising, however, is only one of the many marketing tools in the promotion category.

Most physicians and communication experts believe that, sooner or later, economic pressure will make marketing practices widespread. And as doctors learn that marketing is more than just advertising, their dislike tends to evaporate.

Other Options

Marketing your practice is not the only solution to competition. Other responses to competitive pressures reported by physicians include forming joint ventures with hospitals in developing lower-cost products and services, such as ambulatory care, HMOs, and PPOs, which the hospitals then market to the community.

Many physicians are opting to bypass the headaches of private practice altogether for positions with prepaid health plans and salaries between $35,000 and $50,000: in 1985, 47 percent of physicians under thirty-six years old took such salaried positions, as did 19.4 percent of their older colleagues.[7] The Institute for the Future predicts that by the year 2000, the number of physicians on salary will be nearly double the number on salary in 1988.

By 1997, HMOs will have captured more than 50 percent of the market, predicts Philip Johnston of the Massachusetts Executive Office of Human Services. "HMOs, PPOs, ambulatory surgery centers, docs-in-a-box, all of the newfangled models will dominate, and I think that physicians are going to be radically changed," he says.[8] A report released in Massachusetts in December 1988 indicated that, already, fewer than half that state's physicians work in private offices, with the proportion declining, while the number of physicians practicing in HMOs increased more than five-fold between 1976 and 1988.[9]

These trends do not mean that private medical practice is untenable. Most experts agree that to compete in today's overcrowded marketplace, to assure a healthy patient load for the practice, the solution is good, old-fashioned communication. And a number of physicians are finding that some of the new-fashioned tools, used under the right circumstances, can do wonders for a practice.

Frank Tursi of Erie, Pennsylvania, relates how, with some quick maneuvering, he was able in only a few weeks' time to establish his own long-planned walk-in clinic before a hospital opened a competing one nearby. With the assistance of a public relations expert, he launched a direct marketing campaign, made appearances on local radio and television shows, arranged feature articles, and ran small ads in newspapers. Results were immediate, and the patient census remained strong even during the hospital's marketing blitz when its competing facility opened.

Notes
1. *See* Folland, 311.
2. *See* Steptoe, 1. Reprinted by permission of the *Wall Street Journal*, © Dow Jones & Company, Inc., 1987. All Rights Reserved Worldwide.
3. Hall, 1.
4. *See* Burton, 62.
5. *Ibid.*
6. *See* Hall, 1.
7. *See* Pear, 1.
8. *See* Kiely, 14.
9. Knox, 33.

10 MARKETING, PUBLIC RELATIONS, ADVERTISING: WHAT'S THE DIFFERENCE?

Though frowned upon only a few years ago, marketing by physicians has spread across the country. Starting on the West Coast, it is sweeping down the Sunbelt and heading toward the Northeast corridor, Dr. Andrew Morley of Health Services Marketing, an Atlanta medical marketing firm, told *Physician's Financial News.*[1]

Despite physicians' initial reluctance to add a hard-edged business sense to their medical practices, the rapid and significant changes in the climate for medicine during the last decade have sent many scurrying for prescriptions for ailing practices. Increasing competition, especially, is driving them to consider marketing techniques. In areas with too many doctors, "the average private practitioner is running absolutely scared stiff. His income is down, his patient base is down. He knows darn well that he's got to scramble just to stay even," says Dr. Laurens White, chairman of the board of the California Medical Association.[2]

First embraced by the more consumer-oriented medical specialties of plastic surgery and ophthalmology, which depend heavily on patient self-referrals, marketing has become popular with primary care providers as well, and even with hospital-based physicians seeking to stimulate referrals.

Marketing Is More Than Advertising

To most people who are not aware of its many facets, the word *marketing* means business and a bottom-line orientation, in direct opposition to medicine's service orientation. The most visible aspect of marketing is promotion. Until physicians discover that promotion is only the tip of the marketing iceberg, the part usually used last and least by medical practices, the term *marketing* makes most queasy. But marketing is gaining broader acceptance and understanding among physicians as they discover that its scope is broader than advertising—or being nice to patients, according to Steven W. Brown, past president of the American Marketing Association.[3]

Marketing has emerged as a dominant force in health care, even for those who only a few years ago believed that a business orientation would compromise health care's service mission. Marketing, says public relations expert Nancy Hicks, has become the key to survival.

As American doctors have resorted to creative means of keeping existing patients and luring new ones into their offices in the last few years, marketing, with its patient orientation and its focus on satisfying both patients and physicians, has not only become acceptable but has won the plaudits of a broad range of physicians.

Consultants, too, advocate the use of marketing by medical practices. A marketing strategy is the most important part of a business plan, financial planner Neal Greenberg tells physicians. Learning more about advertising, promotion, and public relations helps doctors become more effective in the marketplace, consultants say.

What is this key to survival all about? What are its elements, its tools, its costs, its relative advantages, and its pitfalls for the fee-for-service medical provider? What role can, does, and should it play in the private practice of medicine?

Health Care Marketing

Because much confusion still exists among health care providers about what marketing is all about, the process is often reduced to the use of a few tools in the hope of a quick fix, overlooking the most essential prescription for success: learning what patients need and want, and responding appropriately. "When people in health care use the word *marketing*, they usually mean the communications part of marketing—promotion or advertising," while ignoring marketing fundamentals like research and strategic planning, says Frank Weaver, director of public affairs at the Cleveland Clinic Foundation.[4]

Ideally, a medical practice with a marketing orientation will determine the needs and wants of patients and attempt to satisfy them through the design, communication, pricing, and delivery of appropriate and competitively viable services, says marketing expert Philip Kotler.[5] However, health care is not yet driven by consumers' true needs, according to Chicago public relations health care specialist Nancy Newman.

Greg Korneluk, a practice management consultant and former program director of the American Medical Association's Department of Practice Management, has defined marketing as "an organized approach to the tasks of planning, pricing, promoting, and delivering your services to patients." It embodies a wide range of activities, with strategies ranging from "very passive and conservative to flamboyant and aggressive."[6]

Other practice management consultants view marketing as a vehicle for practice building, with a focus on patient recruitment as well as recruitment among referring physicians.

Most consultants agree that marketing results in benefits to both doctor and patient. For the physician, the draw is a more stable practice. For the patient, marketing results in better service. "Marketing is a proven methodology that works. It can help you understand your patients better, and, in turn, show you how to motivate and work with them, both for their own benefit and the benefit of your practice," Korneluk has told the physicians who have attended his nationwide seminars.[7]

Marketing Professional Services

People have different expectations of physicians than of other service providers. They expect the physician they select to be adequately trained, to be dedicated to his or her work, and to have up-to-date expertise in his or her specialty. They expect this expertise to be delivered in a manner that inspires trust and confidence, say marketers Doris Van Doren and Louise Smith. Furthermore, because the delivery of professional services is qualitatively different from the delivery of other services, the marketing of professional services differs from the marketing of other services.

The marketing of services, in turn, differs from the marketing of products. The benefits of services are intangible, inconsistent, and inseparable from the deliverer of the service, according to Eric Berkowitz, a marketing professor who has written extensively on health care marketing. In determining the marketing mix for services, the elements of service—pricing, promotion, and even distribution—are different than they are for products, and must be viewed from that unique vantage point. When patients "buy" medical care, which they cannot really judge because of its intangibility, they do not use the "primary product," medical expertise, as a basis for selecting a service provider. Rather, they base their evaluation on the "offered component" of the service: the cost of the visit, the way the office looks, the treatment received from staff, the time it takes to get an appointment. This fact is stressed by medical practice management consultants as well.

"In the minds of most patients, the medical services provided by doctors are identical," Korneluk has written. "A patient generally bases his choice of a physician on other factors: your manner, the convenience of your location, parking availability, the appearance and cleanliness of your office, the attitude of your staff." [8]

A professional service marketer must assess which attributes are most important to patients, keeping in mind that consumers judge services on the tangible evidence provided during their interaction with the doctor and his office staff.

Marketing versus Public Relations

A medical provider seeking professional practice-building help may find it difficult to decide whether a communication, marketing, practice management, public relations, or advertising firm is most suitable for getting the job done. While marketing is the term generally used as the umbrella under which public relations, advertising, and publicity are included, there is often much confusion about where marketing stops and public relations begins, and about the role each plays. Since there are also conflicting views as to whether public relations and marketing are separate but equal functions, equal and overlapping functions, or the same function,[9] an examination of the philosophies of each may prove to be of value.

Marketing reacts to existing needs and wants of patients by developing services that satisfy them. Public relations, on the other hand, is concerned with the attitudes of current and potential patients to a practice, and with cultivating the good will of various publics, including referring physicians. Kotler and Clarke view health care public relations as a part of the marketing mix a medical practice would undertake to pursue its objectives.

While the philosophical orientation of each dictates different responsibilities (market assessment and pricing for marketing; media releases and publications for public relations), there are areas where there are shared responsibilities (see below). There are also tasks common to both, including public surveys, advertising, media strategy, and image assessment, according to Berkowitz. Thus, while both marketing and public relations have their unique aspects, there is some overlap of roles.

Korneluk identifies public relations by its activities, and marketing as the philosophy and management

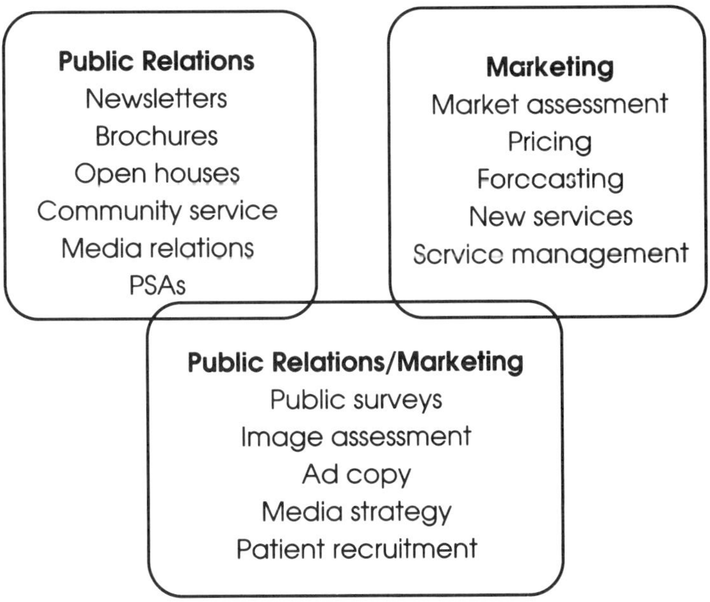

methodology that guides these activities. Thus, public relations indirectly promotes the positive achievements of a practice by the use of news releases, public speaking, and radio and television appearances. He also stresses patient relations as a marketing priority, though generally the latter falls within the purview of public relations.

Perhaps the most relevant distinction has to do with educational backgrounds. Marketers usually train in business schools, stress a profit orientation, and have little exposure to the subjects of communication and mass media. Public relations practitioners, on the other hand, learn communication and media skills and have little training in economics or social analysis, according to Kotler and William Mindak.

It is evident that the distinctions made between marketing and public relations in the health care field are fuzzy at best. Some health care promoters say marketing is the name of the game, whereas others believe the principles of public relations best serve health care providers. Still others say marketing is simply the latest buzzword for what has previously been called patient education and practice management. Making distinctions is no easy task, even for the experts.

While many believe that the principles of public relations work best for health care, they also believe that public relations people working in health care must adopt the mind-set of marketing, broadening their horizons to include research, strategic planning, and other principles of business. However, whether marketing or public relations is *the* important discipline is of little relevance to the physician.

Marketing and public relations professionals in health care are increasingly called upon to promote medical practices using a full-spectrum program that includes elements of marketing, public relations, and sometimes advertising campaigns. The onus is on the marketing, public relations, practice-management, or advertising professional working with physicians to consider the broad range of available tools, much as the physician considers which of the multitude of available medications best treats a patient with a particular ailment.

Cost of Marketing

Cost, always an important consideration, varies widely depending on the scope of services desired, on geographic location, and even on the size of the consulting firm. Experts say that a comprehensive marketing plan can cost up to 5 percent of gross income, but less costly options are available, and at least one consultant, Joyce Sherry, tells physicians to "begin slowly."

Expect to pay from $60 to $125 an hour for your consultant's services. However, consultants generally work on a contractual basis, charging from $1,000 to $2,000 a month, says Chicago-based public relations consultant Julia Schopick.[10] In some areas of the country, fees are much higher. And fees of large firms, reflecting higher overhead costs, tend to be higher than those of smaller ones.

For $3,000 a month for services that typically last from six months to a full year, a California medical marketing/ public relations agency serving solo or small medical group practices conducts a market survey and charts a course of action. Services include basic target audience research, a press kit, news releases, public service announcements, public service fact sheets, physician-referral cards, practice brochures, speakers bureau information, newsletters, and patient billing inserts, all targeted to the physician's local area and designed to be low key. In California, competition is rampant, with doctor-to-patient ratios well above the national norm, and doctors there have found these services, even at $3000 or more per month, worthwhile. On the East Coast, an advertising campaign by two New Jersey surgeons to launch a new service cost $120,000 (see case study, chapter 17).

Practice-management consultants say physicians often come to them after sometimes expensive, often misdirected, do-it-yourself approaches fail. On the flip side, physicians have reported that after working with marketing and public relations consultants and learning marketing techniques, they were able to take over marketing efforts themselves.

Do-It-Yourself Efforts

Although a do-it-yourself strategy can be as costly as hiring a consultant, take up a physician's valuable time, and lack such important resources as media contacts, which are easily reached through the professional medical marketer, physicians who have tried it have found their efforts were rewarded. California dermatologist Donald Hayen and his partner, faced with a shrinking practice, spent $25,000 in the first year of a do-it-yourself campaign that included newsletters, brochures, thank-you notes, *Yellow Pages* display ads, and the hiring of a "practice representative," whose job was to leave brochures, newsletters, and other promotional material with non-physician providers and such area businesses as beauty and nail salons. The doctors found that the increases in both number of patients and income more than compensated for the high cost and the effort involved.

For physicians who want to do their own marketing but lack the know-how, some consultants teach basic strategies, meeting with physicians two to four times a month at a cost in the range of $200 to $500 per month.

Seminars

One-day marketing seminars are available from the American Medical Association in Chicago (at a fee of $195 for AMA members, $245 for nonmembers), from many practice-management consultants who travel around the country, and from state medical associations. The AMA practice marketing seminar provides a workbook for analyzing a practice, setting goals and objectives, selecting target markets, developing a marketing strategy, and monitoring results. The workbook also provides some minimal information about promotional tools. Medical association seminars on marketing, however, have generally attracted sparse audiences, though physicians report having found them useful.

Containing Costs

Hiring a graphic artist to design a logo and develop a new letterhead and color scheme could cost upward of $1,500, but such costs can be contained by hiring graphic arts students and writers from local colleges or universities. Likewise, communication students from local colleges can be hired at a relatively low cost to write copy for brochures and other educational and promotional materials. Hospital public relations staff members have also been hired on a freelance basis by physicians to prepare promotional materials. However, most hospital marketing/public relations staff members, who work long hours and often attend hospital-related events in the evening, may be reluctant to take on additional work.

Notes

1. *See* Wallen 1987, PB1.
2 *See* Burton, 62.
3. *See* Note 1.
4. *See* Hicks, 30.
5. Kotler 1987, 31.
6. Korneluk 1982b, 27.
7. *Ibid.*
8. Korneluk 1982a, 228.
9. *See* Kotler and Clarke, 489.
10. Schopick 1987b, 14. Reprinted with permission from *American Medical News*, © 1987 American Medical Association.

11 PUBLIC RELATIONS: SHAPING PUBLIC ATTITUDES

"Many physicians are doing a lot of public relations without being aware that they are doing it," Edward L. Bernays, the "father of public relations," told me in 1987.

My subsequent research and media reports confirm this. For example, Vermont physicians who are providing free medical care to the indigent are, perhaps without considering their service in such terms, engaging in public relations activities. In general, doctors are willing to work at improving doctor-patient relationships and to undertake patient education and health promotion activities, but they are not likely to refer to or think of these activities as public relations strategies.

Effective public relations has been defined as high quality performance coupled with effective interpretation, the latter requiring that physicians communicate with a diverse and segmented public. Because activities associated with public relations are often considered to have a softer edge than those commonly defined as marketing efforts, they may be more in line with physician values and attitudes and with medicine's traditional service orientation. Physicians may therefore be more inclined to embrace activities traditionally associated with public relations than more aggressive marketing strategies.

The Doctor's Role in Society

According to Julia Schopick, public relations for doctors should mean getting out into their communities and educating the public about their area of expertise. Joining medical societies and writing articles for medical journals serve to communicate only with other physicians, not the public, she says.

Likewise, Edward Bernays urges physicians to be in the forefront of health promotion, a natural extension of their societal role. Other public relations consultants and physicians agree. "I believe it is the obligation of physicians . . . to keep the public informed so that they may understand the moral and social consequences of their actions," Dr. Irvine Page said.

When changes in health care are proposed, the public is more likely to be influenced by the opinions of practicing physicians than by those of government or business groups, according to health analysts. Physicians will *not* contribute effectively to debate by talking only to each other at meetings or in medical journals. The public should become aware of the larger issues, says newspaper editor John Grace.

In 1968, Rex Harlow, then in his fifty-fifth year of a distinguished career in public relations as a consultant, educator, and author, told physicians that their public relations efforts should be directed first to doctor-patient relationships, then to community service, perhaps in conjunction with their county medical societies. By becoming a first-class public relations man, Harlow wrote, the physician "will grow in stature as a man and a citizen. He will win his spurs in public service, take his place as a constructive force in society, contribute to the strength and forward movement of his profession, and enlarge and improve his practice." That is much the same advice being proffered today, but with greater urgency.

Twenty-plus years ago, Harlow's commonsense advice was given in an atmosphere devoid of diagnosis related groups (DRGs), rampant intrusion of third-party interest into the doctor-patient relationship, and scores of physicians frustrated by the replacement of the "art" of medicine with bureaucratic guidelines for medical treatment.

PR Can Help Stem Government Interference

Today, with external forces shaping the attitudes of the public, physicians are being exhorted by their medical societies to make their views public in an effort to stem the tide of distrust that inevitably leads to government intervention, and to explain to the public the potential effect of regulation on the delivery of quality health care.

Public relations activities, with their thrust on patient education, better communication with patients, and publicity, can provide the forum and the public support the medical profession needs to retain its authority and quiet the activist voices rising in protest against doctors perceived as greedy and uncaring.

Senior citizen councils and other organized groups are marching to their legislators' doors and convincing them that doctors need to be regulated. But these same activist groups who begrudge physicians their fees have also clamored for repeal of government regulation of health care, most notably restrictions on hospital stays of Medicare patients resulting from DRGs. Senior citizens could be marching as allies of physicians rather than against them, a more natural alignment of two groups with a long history of common concern for access to and delivery of quality health care.

As Peter Mathieu, former president of the Providence (Rhode Island) Medical Association, has said, "Physicians must band together and let their community hear that physicians do take care of the health needs of the community to the best of their ability, that physicians are available for medical care, and that physicians do worry about their patients and the quality of their service. This effort must be constant, for physicians and patients are equally desirous of a successful health care system."

Mathieu's views are echoed by medical societies across the country. They repeatedly urge physicians to devote some of their time, energy, and money to cope with the public climate and attitude. Yet for decades, physicians have generally relied on their medical associations to perform these public relations tasks.

The Role of Professional Associations

Most national, state, county, and specialty medical associations serve the educational and informational needs of member physicians. In addition, public relations programs are common, aimed at creating a climate of support for members by influencing legislators and evoking a favorable public response. Such programs are frequently planned and executed by public relations experts hired to conduct national public service or public education campaigns that include television, radio, newspaper and magazine materials, PSAs, and other public education materials.

"We must work to capture favorable attention or risk being swept into subjugation by the nature and forces of our times," Vernon Astler told Florida physicians. "We must help create the climate in which we function, rather than let that climate develop and then try to cope or to react to it . . . . While physicians labor in their offices, outside groups and forces are shaping public attitudes which will determine whether physicians will be able to function at all," he warned.

Despite their efforts, many professional medical associations have been accused of being reactive rather than proactive, and doubt has been expressed as to whether they will be able to meet the challenges of the changing world of medicine. Many of the associations, with the exception of the AMA, have been accused of doing little to help physicians prepare for change in their profession.

Yet physicians continue to rely upon and endorse the public affairs activities of their professional organizations. According to recent poll results, physicians overwhelmingly believe that the AMA should continue to take strong positions on public health policies.

But those physicians active in Washington say that to prevent bureaucrats—many of whom may not understand the requirements of good medical care—from making untenable decisions for medicine for which doctors will ultimately bear the blame, more doctors must become actively involved in public affairs. Doctors, says Walter Judd, a physician and former congressman, should work in politics by studying the issues, spreading their views to patients and to the community, and joining a political party. And, if necessary, they should run for office, as he did.

Elected representatives can usually predict the positions of the two major medical lobbies—the American Medical Association and the Association of American Medical Colleges. Congressmen tell physician-lobbyists that they would like to hear more from individual physicians.

The Need for Grassroots Support

Meeting with elected representatives requires a clear message, the skills to deliver that message effectively, and a thorough grounding in the issues to be discussed—work best left to trained spokespersons. However, practicing physicians, as ground troops for their medical societies, can gain the good will of the public—practice by practice and community by community—thereby providing an equally important element of a public relations campaign. Their role is to gain the grassroots support necessary for the accomplishment of associations' political goals. The outcome will influence their own practices in the years ahead.

Toward this goal, medical societies request that their members follow a course of action that establishes confidence in and understanding of the medical profession. This begins with the doctor-patient relationship. Medical public relations places emphasis on the personal human relationship between doctor and patient. According to Harlow, maintaining satisfactory relations with patients calls for a physician's keen appreciation of and skillful use of communication tools and techniques.

Physicians are advised by their medical associations to take the following steps to garner good will for the profession:

- Train ancillary staff to be sympathetic to patients.
- Devote several hours each week to public relations—to Kiwanis appearances, football team exams, immunization programs, and so forth.
- Participate in and support public education programs developed by medical associations—by involving patients in no-smoking days, for instance.
- Learn communications skills.

Whether the goal is to promote public confidence in the profession, to market existing or new services, to establish a new practice, or to maintain a loyal patient base, physicians are being advised to inject a larger dose of two-way conversation into their treatment regimens.

Are doctors prepared to fulfill the communication tasks requested of them by their medical associations? Some no doubt are. But many will need the advice, planning capability, and contacts of public relations professionals as they seek to become more effective communicators. Such advice can be invaluable as physicians step outside their practices into the media spotlight.

12 GETTING MEDIA ATTENTION

Doctors have been spending a lot of time in the news these days. Or rather, the media have been spending a lot of time presenting images of doctors, both real and fictitious. Some of the coverage has been positive, some negative.

Although it is generally recognized that such factors as advances in medical science, societal pressures, and the high cost of health care have all had their impact on the doctor image, many doctors blame the media for portraying physicians unfavorably, thereby tarnishing the profession's image. Media representatives respond by saying doctors pay a price in the media and elsewhere for their affluence and that as a group, their motives, judgment, and competence are being challenged. It is the media's job to expose wrongdoing, inefficiency, and excessive fees charged by some health care providers, just as they point out these wrongdoings in business and government.

Newspaperman Kenneth Byerly tells the story of a colleague who, when speaking to a medical group said, "Half of you probably hate the guts of newspapermen, some tolerate them as a necessary evil, and a few of you may actually like and understand them."

A physician interrupted. "You're wrong," he said, "if you think half of us hate the guts of newspapermen. We all do."

Physicians often point their fingers in frustration at the media, citing hurried reporting, inadequate research, and the lack of medical reporters capable of understanding the complexities of today's medical stories. Nevertheless, many doctors, aware of the need to voice their point of view through the media, advocate a closer relationship between physicians and local news outlets. Some physicians have even given up practice to become full-time media doctors, in order, they say, to provide solid medical reporting to a public clamoring for news relating to medicine and health. The media can be and are being used to shape the climate for medicine. They are also the preferred means of promoting professional services, through publicity.

Physicians in the Limelight

A new publicity trend, that of physician as celebrity, seems to be taking root. Across the country, the life and work of individual physicians have recently been featured in various media outlets—in newspaper and magazine articles, on radio, on television, and on cable programs. *Boston Magazine* recently devoted a thirteen-page article to breast surgeon Susan Love. She has also appeared on two television programs, *NOVA* and *Nightline*.

What physician hasn't wondered what it might be like to be in the limelight? It would be difficult to deny that favorable publicity can have a salutary effect on any medical practice. A physician mentioned in the city magazine of a large metropolitan area as one of the "best internists" in the area is scheduling appointments for new patients nearly two years in the future. Dr. Love has restricted her practice to patients previously diagnosed as having breast cancer. Even then, the wait for an appointment can be lengthy.

Publicity is the domain of public relations professionals, who make much use of this means of promotion. Public relations counselors provide a number of practical suggestions for getting media attention, and for dealing with the media most effectively and ethically.

Attracting Media Attention

One media axiom to know: "The smaller the town, the bigger the news: the bigger the town, the smaller the news." In a small community, just about anything new or unique about the practice stands a good chance of being covered by local media. But adding a new physician to your practice is not material that would interest the *New York Times* or the *Boston Globe.*

The news media in towns large and small, however, are always looking for physicians with some expertise in health-related issues in the news, such as AIDS, new cancer treatments, and so forth. Some pointers on what may interest the media—and how to get involved—follow:

> Watch headlines and news stories for opportunities to contribute your expert advice, opinion, or assistance. A pediatrician might impart information on hazardous toys or other safety issues prior to the Christmas season; a dermatologist might prepare an article on preventing sun damage; an internist or family practitioner might want to comment on the increased use of steroids by teenagers. Trends, seasons, national weeks and months, all provide fodder for newsworthy stories.

Visibility through the media is best suggested by a middleman—usually a public relations person—lest it be construed as grandstanding on the physician's part.

After the media introductions have been made, however, calls to newspaper, television, or radio editors about newsworthy items should be made personally. An editor who is interested in a story idea may want to ask the physician more questions on the spot.

Keep calls to editors and reporters short and succinct. Media personnel work under difficult deadlines. If you call a newspaper, it may be wise to time your call for after the day's edition "goes to bed."

Take a stand on medical issues in the news, and make that stand known by writing letters to the editor, which may appear on the op-ed page of your local newspaper.

Offer to be an ongoing consultant in medicine to local newspapers and radio or television stations—preferably through an intermediary.

Offer to appear on television or radio call-in "Ask the Doctor" type shows. Cable programming also allows opportunities to appear on local health shows.

Volunteer to do public service announcements for your local hospital or medical society.

Volunteer to write a health column for your local newspaper or to answer readers' health questions. But if you do, make sure you have time to undertake this project and that you are capable of meeting the deadlines. No time? Some physicians hire public relations firms or freelance medical writers to ghostwrite and place articles in newspapers and magazines.

Submit articles to your local newspapers on events surrounding your practice: openings, open houses, new staff members, new equipment procurements.

If your practice is making news—a new procedure, a new treatment, a prestigious award or appointment to one of the physicians—ensure that the information will be reported accurately by distributing a news release.

For the print media, the news item should be typed on your stationery. On top, at the left margin under your letterhead, type FOR IMMEDIATE RELEASE so that the media know they can use the material immediately. On the same line, in the center, type CONTACT:______with the name of the physician to be contacted and both *day and evening* telephone numbers for the person listed.

For television, a news release should be short—about ninety seconds maximum. Keep in mind when planning the script that it could be aired any time within sixty days after release, and avoid mentioning specific days or dates. Use five-minute, three-quarter-inch tape cassettes. Send the tape to the producer (only if he or she has been contacted previously and has expressed interest) in a clearly marked package for easy identification.

Use audiocassettes for radio news releases. They too should be short, usually thirty seconds. Sixty seconds is the maximum. Send the tape in a clearly marked package to a producer or editor who has expressed interest.

The following are appropriate opportunities to send releases to local news outlets: upon return from a seminar/course you have attended to learn a new procedure or therapy; upon publication of an article in a clinical journal; when participating in scheduled lectures or programs; when you have achieved certification or membership in a specialty society; if you have been elected to a status position by a local civic, religious, social, or sports group; and if you have received a teaching appointment.

Don't play favorites by giving your information to only one reporter: contact all appropriate news outlets simultaneously. Unless there is a very good reason to give an "exclusive" to one reporter, don't.

If you are going to contact media people, inform your staff that they may be returning your calls.

Return calls to the media promptly if you want to be the expert quoted. Ask your staff to alert you when the media call rather than to leave a message you may not see until the end of the day. If you are tied up with an emergency or in the O. R. when a reporter calls, return the call as promptly as you can.

Have an acceptable, flattering photograph of each member of your group on hand. Newspapers use black and white photos. Color slides are appropriate for the broadcast media.

Make It Newsworthy

"New and different" are the keys to enticing the media, and Don Kirkland of Health Services Marketing suggests that physicians go through the following self-questioning process prior to submitting any story suggestion to the media:

- Does it represent a new way of treating a common medical condition?
- Does it illustrate a particularly positive outcome in a case in which a positive outcome isn't normally expected?

- May it have an impact on the way patients with similar conditions are treated in the future?

Kirkland also suggests that news stories with errors be handled diplomatically. Minor errors should be ignored. If the error cannot be ignored, call the reporter involved, but try to avoid use of the word *retraction*, which has the same effect on a reporter as the word *malpractice* has on a physician. If the matter cannot be resolved with the reporter, then write a *short* letter to the editor indicating that the reporter has confused the issue or misstated facts.

Establishing Good Working Relations with the Media

To establish good working relations with the media, consultants suggest the following:

Get to know local medical and health editors.

Prepare the press for upcoming medical stories by distributing background information and guiding reporters to the most important articles in medical journals.

Stage seminars for the press at which complex medical topics are discussed—in lay language, of course.

If you are approached by a reporter after a scientific meeting, be patient and take the time to clarify everything the reporter doesn't understand.

Don't demand that an article be written exactly as you give it. However, you can insist that direct quotes not be altered.

Don't argue with a reporter—an article about you

that began favorably may end up with an unexpectedly negative twist.

If you are unsure of a position or need more information, tell the reporter you'll get back to him or her as soon as possible. Ask what the reporter's deadline is and respect it, leaving the reporter some leeway for writing up the information you provide.

Keep in mind that nothing turns the press off more than unfulfilled promises to return a call.

Send a note of appreciation to the reporter for good work. It pays off.

When to Get Expert Advice

Publicity can make or break a professional reputation. It is one area in which an expert's advice can prove invaluable. Just as you wouldn't expect to treat a patient without the knowledge and experience to do the job, so you shouldn't expect to handle public communication without some training and practice.

From the media's perspective, doctors make poor sources for medical stories. In a study of newspapers, network news broadcasts, and wire service reports on a medical topic—an influenza inoculation campaign—Rubin and Hendy found that journalists did not regard physicians as good sources. Virtually none of the journalists contacted private physicians for information. Instead, they relied on official government sources such as the Center for Disease Control. Their reasons? Journalists said that, as sources, doctors ranged from "lousy" to tellers of half truths trying to protect an image. They cited also the unwillingness of doctors to publicly state views that were in opposition to those held by the medical establishment.

Dale Carnegie, in his famous book *Public Speaking*

wrote: "I remember hearing a physician say in a talk that 'diaphragmatic breathing is a distinct aid to peristaltic action of the intestines, and a boon to health.'" Carnegie stopped the speaker and asked the lay audience for a show of hands from those who understood what the physician had said. No hands were raised.

Unless you have a background in communication, some media training focusing on how to present your story to the media is highly desirable. Trained in communication skills and armed with media contacts, public relations consultants can arrange media appearances and prepare physicians for them. Many public relations firms teach physicians how to communicate effectively in the media. Through individual instruction and videotape critiques, they allow physicians to see themselves as others see them. Communication experts know what it takes to get a message across, and how to do it most effectively.

For physicians who want to obtain initial media attention, hiring a consultant is the usual route. Given the media's skepticism about physicians, the chances of being chosen to be a media health consultant are greater if the request is made by a communication expert than by a physician.

Important Considerations Regarding Publicity

If you have the opportunity to appear on a television or radio program, to write a column or an article, or to be the subject of a feature, remember that the media should be used as a vehicle to promote health rather than to create celebrity for an individual physician, even if the stated goal is to boost the practice. With preparation and knowledge of how the media operate, physicians can effectively position themselves as experts in their specialties. This can build a practice while protecting the reputation of the profession.

On medical issues of public concern, such as the ramifications of the high cost of malpractice insurance or the quality of health care provided by HMOs, initiative in dealing with the media is important. Act, don't react, consultants advise. The first story on any issue often has the greatest impact, and physicians must begin to get their side of the story out first. However, prompt, factual responses to medical issues already in the news are also important and encouraged by both communication consultants and organized medical associations.

Television and radio talk show appearances are not the only methods of obtaining publicity, though they are the most visible. Community speaking engagements and articles written for local newspapers and magazines can also position a physician as an expert in his field. Another route to being considered an expert is to write a book.

Publicity falls within the more aggressive communication category. To be effective, it should follow rather than precede a sound patient relations program. Publicity without sound public relations is not worth very much. Without good service in the office, publicity is useless. All the publicity in the world won't generate a thriving practice for a physician perceived by patients to be uncaring or incompetent.

For several reasons, publicity as a means of practice promotion is desirable. It puts a physician's name before the public and helps to attract new patients, it is more acceptable than advertising, and it is free. The most desirable publicity is that which positions a physician as an expert in his specialty.

But prior to committing the time to participate in high-visibility patient education or health promotion activities, a physician should ask himself or herself:

> Will participation in this fair or giving this talk allow me the opportunity to discuss topics at which I am particularly skilled?

Will it help position me as an expert in my field?

Will providing free screenings generate the type of publicity that enhances my practice?

Perils and Pitfalls to Avoid

Not every physician can promote a practice successfully by appearing on a talk show, and not every mention in the press is good public relations. Physicians who can benefit most from publicity are those who can speak effectively without using medical jargon, enjoy educating people, and understand what can be publicized about their specialities or practices.

Publicity has its risks. The media can exploit naive physicians into giving scoops on medical "breakthroughs" which overpromise and, in the long run, erode the public image of physicians further. Conversely, some physicians have earned the disdain of their peers and the public by using the media to promote themselves instead of viewing publicity in its proper perspective—as an educational tool to achieve the broader goal of patient or community education about health issues.

At least one medical association has warned its members that reporters' objectives are in direct conflict with the medical profession's long-established policy of depersonalized reporting and avoidance of unfair personal aggrandizement. Reporters look for the spectacular, the glamorous, and the bizarre: dignified, circumspect, and objective information makes poor press. The danger: a naive physician who agrees to appear on television to discuss a medical point may find himself in the hot seat. Be prepared.

The following are tips on some of the dangers and how to avoid them:

In your effort to be helpful to the media, don't rush into making a public statement before you have had a chance to prepare a statement, rehearse it, and examine it carefully for possible problems. Ask yourself, could this be misconstrued?

If you feel that a ten-minute interview on the phone will not do justice to a complex topic, invite the reporter to your office for a more thorough demonstration.

When talking to the media, establish up front whether your statements are for publication or "off the record." Even so, though most journalists will respect your position, the rule of thumb is, "If you don't want to see it in print, don't say it."

Be aware that reporters look for diversity of opinion. If a reporter is digging for information that you are unwilling to discuss or prefer not to handle, such as commenting about another physician's work, don't be evasive. Say, "I'd rather not comment on that at this time," and refer the reporter to your hospital's public relations director, who is trained to handle such situations (and tell the PR person to expect the call).

Remember that you are under no obligation to speak to a reporter. First assess, via the local hospital public relations department, the reputation of the reporter, the editor, and the newspaper or program. Then ask:

- Who is asking for the interview?
- What is the publication?
- Why do they want it?
- What's the angle of the story?
- What information do they already have?
- Who else are they talking to?

- What do I get out of it?

For a physician interested in taking the publicity route, the first stop for advice should be to the public relations, marketing, or communication department of the local hospital.

13 PREPARING FOR RADIO AND TELEVISION APPEARANCES

A radio interview or television appearance is a prime opportunity to gain exposure, convey a message, and achieve recognition. Preparation is the key to a successful interview. No performer would make a stage appearance to speak before hundreds, perhaps millions of people without training and at least some rehearsal. Physicians, too, need preparation before they sit in front of the cameras and microphones.

You have to know what you are going to say, how to get your message across, and, for television, how to dress. On television the way you look and act may be more important than what you actually say. Following are interview tips by experts who prepare physicians, businessmen, and other professionals for electronic media appearances.

Do Your Homework

Ask in advance how much ground the interview will cover. Is the interviewer interested in a representative opinion or in your personal views? Are details relating to your own practice or your specialty of prime interest?

Learn the interviewer's angle, who else will be on the program, and what information the interviewer already has.

Determine whether the interview is to be closed or open. Will the interviewer seek factual information on a specific topic (closed) or pursue a general line of questioning (open) and depend on you to develop ideas and direction?

Be informed and as sure of your facts as possible. On television, you will not be able to use note cards.

Listen to or watch the show several times prior to your appearance. Observe the interviewer, listening for the types of questions he or she asks.

Set objectives you want to accomplish, and prepare "mini-speeches" you can bridge into when there is an opportunity to do so. Rehearse these, but not so much that your remarks sound canned.

Visual aids add interest to an interview format because they take the focus off "talking heads" and often help to illustrate a point or a procedure. If you will be using them, check with the producer and director beforehand on size and appropriate colors. Visual aids are either horizontal, glass-mounted slides or three-quarter-inch videotapes.

Provide the interviewer with a list of frequently asked questions about your subject prior to your appearance.

Anticipate questions, especially challenging or embarrassing ones, and prepare responses.

Be ready to respond to an embarrassing quote from your past. Assume that the interviewers have done *their* homework.

Have in mind an overall objective—the most important point you want to make, for example.

Dressing for Television

Both men and women should wear their glasses if they normally do so.

Men

Choose a suit in a medium color: gray, blue, brown, or mixtures. Very dark clothing, such as navy blue, black, or dark brown, tends to lose its detail, so stick to the medium shades. Avoid stripes, checks, and very fine patterns.

Gray or light blue shirts give the best effect, but other light or pastel colors also work well. Pure white shirts may be worn but are not generally recommended, as they may present lighting problems to the studio.

Choose a necktie with a fairly large pattern, in a darker color than your shirt. Don't wear a bow tie, which tends to move when you speak and may distract the viewer from your message.

Wear over-the-calf socks to avoid having your ankles show when you cross your legs. Socks and trousers should match.

Pocket handkerchiefs are *not* recommended. If you must wear one, choose a solid color that complements your suit. Have someone look in the monitor to make sure it appears straight and looks well pressed.

Do not wear highly polished tie clasps or cuff links. They cause flaring and distortion of the television picture.

Use makeup to avoid skin shininess. If you have a dark beard, a high forehead, or a receding hairline, makeup is especially necessary. Dust a corn silk "non-color" powder over makeup to even out the color and reduce shiny spots. The television crew can supply professional makeup.

Women

Wear clothes that provide good contrast for your face and hands. Solid colors are best. Patterns, particularly finely detailed ones, may make you appear to ripple across the screen.

Do not wear large pieces of highly polished jewelry. They can cause glare.

Use your regular makeup. If you don't routinely wear makeup, use a corn silk "non-color" pressed powder to reduce your skin's normal shininess.

Wear dark shoes.

Facing the Camera

Before Going on the Air

Arrive early. If possible, look at the set before the interview. Establish rapport with the host, and decide how you will address each other on camera.

Check in the mirror to make sure your clothing is hanging properly. Remove your wallet, glasses, keys, and other bulky items from your pockets.

Calm jittery nerves and relax your throat muscles by yawning or stretching.

Review your material. Don't be afraid to walk around the studio talking to yourself, reviewing the points you're planning to make.

Tell yourself that you're glad to be there, you're interested in the audience, and you're an authority on the subject matter.

On the Air

If you are seated in a regular chair, turn it at a slight angle toward the interviewer.

If you are seated in a swivel chair, do not swivel. It makes you look uneasy and detracts from your credibility.

Sit up straight and lean slightly toward the interviewer. This gives you the appearance of authority, alertness, and interest in the interview.

If you are interviewed standing up, stand straight. The interviewer will place the microphone. Don't look at or touch it. Keep your hands at your sides, clasped in front of you, or behind your back. Do not fold your arms.

Always look at the interviewer, not the camera. When others are speaking, look directly at them. Don't stare blankly into space.

Never look away from the set, no matter what is going on. There is a great deal of movement in a television studio throughout tapings and broadcasts. Also, resist the temptation to look at yourself on the studio monitor.

Keep your facial expressions neutral. Never frown. Smile when that is appropriate, as when something humorous occurs.

Use your nervousness as energy to express excitement and enthusiasm.

Use hand gestures when you speak, but sparingly. Be natural, as if you were talking to a good friend.

Do not throw your arms over the chair back, or cross and uncross your legs.

Keep your demeanor pleasant. Don't appear argumentative, and never lose your temper, no matter how unpleasant the interviewer.

Be yourself. You are not an actor or actress. Speak in a normal, conversational tone of voice. Never shout.

Speak the way people do in conversation—in short sentences, using easy-to-understand words.

Keep what you say simple. Do not use medical jargon. If you must use a medical term, explain it. Remember, you are speaking to a general audience.

Avoid "um's" and "uh's," "you know," and repeatedly clearing your throat. Instead of using such nonwords, pause. Your pause will give listeners an opportunity to think about what's been said.

Don't try to say too much too fast.

Be concise. The broadcast media are highly capsulized. You may be given only a few seconds to make your point. The average quote on the news is five to ten seconds long. In an interview, no answer should be longer than forty to sixty seconds.

Take the initiative in the conversation occasionally.

Sometimes several questions are asked at once. If that happens, respond to the one you want most to answer.

Don't pretend to be an expert outside of your specialty. Label a question falling outside your area of expertise as such and tactfully decline to respond. If you don't know, say so, and prepare two or three graceful ways to say "I don't know," such as, "That's a question best answered by a cardiac surgeon." Avoid saying "No comment."

Don't volunteer more information than you would like

to give. A trick sometimes used by interviewers is a long pause. If you can refrain from filling it, the interviewer will be forced to go on to other areas.

Don't ask, "Does that answer your question?" at the end of your response.

Listen carefully to the interviewer. Be on the alert for questions that are repeated. Give the same answer the second time around as you did the first time the question was asked.

Don't rush to answer a question. Think your answer through, even while the camera is rolling. You can buy time by asking the interviewer to define a word he's used, by asking for clarification, or by asking for the question to be repeated. Or you can rephrase the question yourself and answer your own, rather than the interviewer's, question.

In the face of hostility, confine yourself to your area of expertise.

If you are asked a troublesome question that is of a general nature, answer only a specific part of the question. On the other hand, if you are asked a hostile specific question, give a more general answer.

Deal with unjustified allegations first if a two-part question is posed.

Don't let yourself get cornered into answering yes or no to a complex question.

Follow a particular question that makes you look bad with a transition to a subject you are confident about.

If you don't want something aired, don't say it, even if you think you're off the air. Because television is a visual medium that requires movement to keep the viewer's interest, the camera operator may unmount the camera and walk around the interview room for cutaways—pictures taken from different angles for variety. Even when the camera is being moved, assume the microphone is still on.

Remain seated until you are told that the interview has ended and that you may leave.

14 HIRING A CONSULTANT

Doctors who hire professional consultants are making more money—23 percent more—than their colleagues who don't, a *Medical Economics* survey found. Even those physicians who spoke to a consultant only once earned 12 percent more.

Apparently, seeking out practice consultants is becoming more common. One of every four physicians reported having used a consultant within the past two years, compared with fewer than one in five in the years 1976–1978.[1]

If a practice is in trouble or a physician needs to hone skills for a television appearance, professional help may be sought. Physicians also use consultants to help boost practice income, improve personnel relations, and to secure management and financial advice. Some have hired consultants to help them reshape their practices to better suit their lifestyles (see chapter 15). And in growing numbers, doctors are hiring experts to promote their practices, to prepare written and audiovisual materials, and to train them and their staffs in communication skills.

Consultants' Services

Medical consultants offer a variety of services, including:

- Practice assessment
- Developing a marketing strategy
- Studying the competition
- Practice-building planning
- Investigating problems and potential solutions
- Image building
- Office staff training
- Preparation of educational, promotional, and advertising materials
- Obtaining publicity
- Identifying and developing new services and markets
- Career planning

Options

Physicians who decide to market their practices have several options. They can adopt a do-it-yourself approach, perhaps with the assistance of a one-day seminar. Those who find that they have neither the time, the inclination, the know-how, nor the staff to market their own practices have other avenues they can explore. One is to hire a consultant who has a knowledge of marketing and the media contacts to do the whole job. The other option is to hire a consultant to help plan and supervise, leaving the implementation of a program to the physician and his or her staff. Physicians can also seek assistance from their medical associations and hospitals.

Medical Association Assistance

The AMA's Department of Practice Management provides a number of workshops, publications, and audiovisual materials aimed at enhancing individual medical practices. Current offerings include the following:

Patient Relations Pack. The three items in the pack, "Winning Ways with Patients," "Preparing a Patient Information Booklet," and "Talking with Patients," aim at improving doctor-patient relations.

Patient Survey Questionnaire. Useful for measuring satisfaction of patients with different aspects of the practice, ranging from office appearance to the whys and wherefores of how patients select a physician.

Market Area Profile Service (MAP). A detailed survey of demographics and other medical services in the area of interest. Includes information on population, number and size of households, per capita income, unemployment rate, number and age of area physicians, number of specialists, number of hospitals, and description of services. According to the AMA, the report is particuarly helpful to physicians investigating new sites or comparing several sites, and for physicians planning to expand or modify services. The area profiled by the MAP service can be a county, city, zip code, group of zip codes, or "ring study," a circular area of any number of miles surrounding a user-specified central point.

Workshop: "Marketing Strategies for Private Practice."

A full-day workshop designed to aid physicians in positioning their practices.

Workshop: "The Competitive Edge: Practice Building Techniques for Today's Health-Care Market." A half-day workshop focusing on techniques in attracting and retaining patients.

Some workshops are held in cities throughout the country, others only at the AMA's Chicago headquarters. Scheduling and price information is available from the American Medical Association, 535 North Dearborn Street, Chicago, IL 60610, (312) 645-5000.

Many state medical associations also have communication, marketing, or practice-management departments that offer services and products designed to help physicians with their marketing and communication needs.

Hospital Assistance

Hospitals, seeking to encourage physicians to fill empty beds at their facilities, have become increasingly active in providing marketing assistance to physicians in the last several years. Hospitals large and small are increasing their physician marketing budgets. In 1988, physician marketing activities increased by some 83 percent, with the average hospital budgeting $24,300 for physician marketing, in the range of $7,900 per year by small hospitals to $110,000 per year by large hospitals. Assistance provided by hospitals includes practice-building programs, physician referral services, and training programs for physicians' office staffs.

Why are hospitals expending funds to help physicians? Sixty-one percent of the three hundred hospital executives surveyed said physician marketing improves the image of their hospitals.[2] By lending a helping hand to their physicians, hospitals as well as physicians benefit: hospitals retain the physicians on staff, and the physicians' practices get a boost.

Physicians Seek Support

Practice-management consultant William Trombetta suggests that hospitals, in the course of seeking mutually beneficial relationships with physicians, will supply physicians with the valuable information required to assess the health of their practices—the type of information upon which marketing consultants rely.

Many physicians have expressed interest in acquiring such data from hospitals. Of five hundred physicians surveyed by the National Research Corporation, 41 percent said they would increase admissions to hospitals that provided practice management and marketing assistance. Of the six categories in which hospitals could assist physicians—marketing, patient care, services, facility/equipment, practice management, and cost containment—marketing was the single largest category of assistance requested. Some 28 percent of the physicians polled said they could use marketing support, including advertising, public relations, and referral services. Preparation of brochures, videotapes, health newsletters, and other patient-directed communications were cited by physicians as the type of marketing support they most wanted.

When asked more specifically about their practice-management needs, physicians found patient relations of greatest interest, with assistance in training office staff desired. Thirty-four percent of the doctors rated patient relations assistance from hospitals as "very valuable," with an additional 42 percent rating it "somewhat important."[3]

Physicians also find hospital-sponsored physician referral programs, the most common form of assistance offered by hospitals, valuable. When hospitals promote physicians through a hospital-sponsored physician-referral program or by including physicians in hospital promotional materials, the advantages to the physician are cost (free), credibility (high), and convenience. Accordingly, in a survey of ten thousand doctors, referral was the preferred hospital service (requested by 67.9 percent of doctors), followed by continuing medical education of office nurses (59.9 percent) and training office staff on guest relations (57.5 percent).[4]

Cable Television

Some hospitals are using cable television to promote the capabilities of their facilities and the physicians on their staffs. Jean Connor, director of corporate communications at Salem Hospital in Massachusetts, produces a monthly show, *Focus on Health*. Each fifteen-to-thirty-minute program is repeated forty-four times during the month in ten different cities and towns in the Salem area. The hospital runs ads in local papers to alert viewers to upcoming programs. The ideal program, Connor says, features two physicians and a patient willing to tell about his or her experience. One such program on children of cancer patients caught the interest of the Public Broadcasting System, which will give an expanded version of the program national exposure.

Other Hospital Programs

Many hospitals have speakers bureaus, which carefully place physicians in contact with groups interested in their specialty. Hospital public relations departments often send out news releases when physicians on their staffs are elected to positions of importance in local, state, or national medical societies. Some hospitals go further, providing full-scale marketing programs for physicians on their staffs, either using in-house staff or hiring outside marketing/public relations consultants to assist physicians. In some cases, the hospital and the physician share the approximately $3,000 cost of a marketing package prepared by an outside firm for the physician.[5]

Despite the assistance available from hospitals, many physicians prefer to hire an outside consultant in order to maintain their privacy. Most doctors don't want to divulge such sensitive items as their income to members of the hospital staff.

How Consultants Differ

My study comparing the approaches of practice-management, public relations, marketing, and advertising consultants in promoting medical practices found that as groups, these consultants varied considerably in their orientation. *Practice-management* consultants gave priority to doctor-patient relations, while *public relations* consultants stressed community service. *Marketing* consultants were equally divided between doctor-patient relations and patient education/health promotion.

These findings are not surprising in light of the fact that public relations consultants seek publicity for their clients, which often coincides with community service. Likewise, practice-management consultants, who are often called in to train staff, to correct office problems, and to increase efficiency, tend to be patient oriented and focus on doctor-patient relations. Marketers, who have patient needs and wants in mind in an effort to create new services or improve existing ones, are also less likely to focus on community activities.

However, the study also found that in the promotion of the professional services of physicians, what consultants call themselves does not necessarily imply use of a stringently defined set of tools. Rather, the use of a variety of tools is common, particularly by practice-management and public relations consultants.

A physician shopping for assistance in promoting his or her practice should look beyond the name of a firm and consider instead its sensitivity to the particular needs, norms, and nuances of promoting a medical practice. Consultants should be chosen who are aware that the practice of medicine is a service devoted to the health of patients, and that this service orientation is in keeping with the norms of the majority of physicians.

Choosing a Consultant

Consultants can be found in practice-management, public relations, marketing, communication, and advertising firms. What they call themselves is less important than their track records in understanding the nature of medical practice and their ability to provide a broad range of marketing options. A referral from another physician is one good guide to choosing a consultant.

Listen for All 4 Ps

A reputable consultant is not likely to recommend a quick fix to practice problems. Rather, he or she will help devise both short-term and long-term strategies for improving your particular situation. Listen for the inclusion of the four Ps of marketing: **p**roduct (your service), **p**ositioning, **p**romotion, and **p**rice (your fee). A consultant who mentions only one of these may be too restricted in scope to plan a successful communication strategy for a medical practice.

Look for a firm or individual who is familiar with the process. Planning based on research is the foundation of any communication effort. The research usually involves questionnaires, telephone surveys, interviews with current and prospective patients, or focus groups. Be wary of any consultant who skips this step.

After research reveals the opportunities available to the practice, the second step involves positioning the practice to take advantage of these. Sometimes this entails improving or revamping the services offered. But if a consultant suggests making major changes in either services offered or target audiences, make sure the suggestions are backed by solid evidence. Also be sure to verify that the outcome will be in line with your own goals for the practice.

Promotion can range from conservative to aggressive. Look for a consultant who has experience in the range you are interested in.

Price is not yet a major factor in choosing a physician, though trends show it is likely to become one (see chapter 16). Unless the majority of your practice serves those age groups most sensitive to fees (adults over 65 and under 35), price should not be given undue weight in the overall plan at this time. It is, however, important to know what other physicians in the area are charging for their services. If your fees are not way off base for your area, be wary of a consultant who stresses price.

Since medicine differs from almost any other type of service, it takes a firm or consultant with some experience and sensitivity to market a medical practice effectively. Firms inexperienced in the health field may recommend actions or promotional activities out of keeping with your own and the profession's philosophy, which may ultimately hurt rather than improve the referral base.

Further Hints on Hiring

The following tips may be helpful in the process of selecting a consultant:

Set your own goals first. Prior to hiring an agency or an individual, determine what you would like to gain from a marketing program and write down your goals.

Look for a consultant who maps out a strategy with the twin objectives of long-term personal satisfaction and financial success.

Get referrals from other physicians in your area, or seek firms that have established a reputation in health care marketing.

Seek a firm or independent consultant with experience working with physicians in your practice size and practice specialty, or with such other health care providers as hospitals and clinics.

Interview firms or independent consultants. Ask about their background, experience, services, and philosophy.

Find out specifically who will be working with you—whether the owner of the agency or an employee—and that person's background, experience, and philosophy on marketing a medical practice.

If several options are available, compare rates, services, and attitudes toward your particular specialty.

Get a written proposal on the services to be provided and their cost. Or decide ahead of time the amount you can afford to spend on a program and request bids in that price range.

Review samples of each firm's work and decide which ones best fit the image and philosophy you would like to present.

Notes
1. *See* Norman, 51.
2. *See* "Physician Marketing . . .," 32.
3. *See* Jensen 1987a, 130.
4. *See* Note 2.
5. *See* Super 1987, 57.

15 RESHAPING AN UNREWARDING CAREER

Disillusioned with medical practice and disheartened by its effects on their lives, many physicians are leaving medicine without considering another option, namely, reshaping their practices to reflect their own personalities and lifestyles, their personal as well as their professional goals.

Reasons for Disillusionment

The loss of public esteem, the declining image, the erosion of autonomy, and doubt regarding future prospects have led to what the *Wall Street Journal*, under the heading "Sad Symptoms of Changing American Medicine," has dubbed the "disaffected doctor" syndrome. This condition, and its causes, have been chronicled by the press over the past several years. The *New York Times* cited "A Squeeze on Doctors' Profits: Even the Group Practices Have Been Hurt by Medicare Rules, High Costs and New Competition." A *Washington Post* headline read, "The Price of Malpractice: How the Crisis Harms the Relationship Between Doctors and Patients." Another *Wall Street Journal* article's front-page headline read, "Hassles and Red Tape Destroy Joy of the Job for

Many Physicians," with the subhead, "Younger Practitioners Quit and Older Ones Retire." Then it asked, "Are the Gripes Sour Grapes?"

This article, letters to the editor prompted by it, and other reports by physicians give many reasons for their disgruntlement. The following quotes by doctors, culled from these sources, are representative of the feelings and concerns of physicians today.

> A growing number of physicians are losing their enthusiasm for medicine, a disaffection that in some way will affect the care every one of us receives. It is a malaise that has spread over the majority of the middle-aged physicians I know. This disaffection is a national tragedy. Rapidly, and to the delight of fools, a health-care system is being altered that since World War II has delivered better health to more people in less time than any system in history. The system, of course imperfect, is properly being modified . . . . Reasonable physicians—and they are in the majority—agree with many of the modifications. But is the discouragement and disillusionment of responsible doctors a necessary consequence of appropriate changes? I submit it is not.[1]

> This problem is urban, suburban and rural. It exists in major teaching institutions and small towns. It affects the national and local medical establishments as well as solo practitioners.[2]

> Once being a doctor was a noble profession. But in the last years, it became just a job.[3]

> It is enormously stressful . . . to feel constant pressure from the conflicting demands of integrating profit-making business practices with consummate professionalism. The challenge to America's doctors is to remain true to their professional ideals in the face of current economic and legal pressures

> and at the same time respond to patients' wishes that they become more caring and sensitive to those same people who lead a "revolt" against them.[4]

> For the first time in 2,000 years of medicine, physicians will be the messengers who will have to say to the sick and injured that the resources are not available to treat every patient with every modern available therapy. There is not enough for everyone.[5]

> Those of us in small, primary care practices may be forced out of business.[6]

Research by the University of Illinois corroborates reports that the demoralization of America's doctors is widespread.[7] And in annual AMA surveys, the last several years are noteworthy for the increase in the variety of problems reported by physicians. These surveys also confirm the feeling among physicians of a continuing loss of autonomy. In response to a question of control over patient treatment, 54 percent of physicians said they felt their autonomy had decreased during the last several years. Most affected were general practitioners (63%), surgeons (62%), psychiatrists (59%), and obstetricians/gynecologists (58%). The 1987 AMA survey found that physicians also reacted strongly against insurance plan provisions requiring that their decisions be reviewed by non-physicians.

Results of Widespread Demoralization

That physicians are giving more than just lip service to their disillusionment is evident from their actions. More young doctors are quitting their practices. Middle-aged and older doctors are switching careers or retiring early. In Illinois, where a physician-owned and -operated company insures about half the state's sixteen thousand practicing doctors, retirements among those insured by the company rose 96 percent over a six-month period compared with the year before. In some states, informal polls by medical societies show that as many as 17 percent of doctors recently decided to retire early, leave medicine, or make serious changes in their practices.

On the national level, the Physician Executive Management Center, which counsels doctors who want to switch to other careers, reported that the number of doctors seeking its advice quadrupled in the past five years. Likewise, the American Academy of Medical Directors, an organization of physicians involved in the business of health care management, reported that its ranks swelled from four hundred in 1984 to twenty-five hundred in 1987. And the Association of American Medical Colleges reports that the number of medical school applicants dropped 37 percent nationwide between 1974 and 1988 as word of disillusionment has spread. Medical education is becoming something of a buyer's market, and some medical schools in Texas and Ohio have, for the first time, begun advertising for students. Others are gearing up to pitch medicine as a career.[8] The *Wall Street Journal* reported that in a survey of twelve hundred students who scored well on the Medical Colleges Admissions Test but didn't apply to medical school, one-fourth said that a physician had discouraged them.[9]

Other Factors in the Exodus

External factors are also causing changes in the practice of fee-for-service medicine. A number of medical specialties are deeply affected by rising malpractice insurance premiums. According to the American College of Obstetrics and Gynecology, one-eighth of its eighteen thousand members dropped the obstetrics side of their practice in 1985, a rise of 37 percent since 1983.

The political climate is having an impact on the practice of medicine in some states. According to the Massachusetts Medical Society, 20 percent of the state's orthopedic surgeons left their practices, prompting the organization to take the unusual step of alerting the medical societies of the forty-nine other states that the political and economic climate in Massachusetts makes it an inhospitable place to practice medicine.

Observers outside the medical field are also noting the changes and their effect on physicians. Says Nathan Hershey, a lawyer and author of a book on hospital-physician relationships, "Many physicians believe—and there is evidence to support their belief—that the private entrepreneurial practice of medicine is on an irreversible downward course and they no longer will be their own masters."

"I can't remember a time when there's been more discomfort and soul-searching," Arnold Relman, who tours the country speaking to physician groups, told the *Wall Street Journal.*[10]

Marketing as a Career Tool

Career neglect apparently can take its toll on physicians' attitudes toward their work and their patients and can affect their overall satisfaction; and it may explain in part the "disaffected doctor" syndrome. In a survey of 754 physicians by publisher Harcourt Brace Jovanovich, 37.5 percent said they would switch careers if a viable alternative presented itself, and only 50 percent said they felt medicine afforded them a desirable lifestyle.

According to some medical marketing consultants, physicians with stable practices but waning interest make the best candidates for a practice makeover; the long-range view dictates a close look at a practice as a reflection of the personality, interests, and career goals of the physician. They also counsel that highly personalized marketing strategies can turn a dull practice into a rewarding career.

Intraprofession Career Changes

American Medical News has reported several cases in which marketing strategies have been successfully employed to make medical practice more rewarding psychologically as well as financially.[11]

As one example, a Michigan plastic surgeon in his late forties left a successful medical practice he no longer enjoyed to attend law school. After passing the bar exam he realized that he was a better doctor than lawyer. He returned to medicine, but not to his previous practice. With the help of a marketing consultant, he tailored a more challenging, satisfying career in cosmetic surgery. The new practice was based on elective surgery, which provided a more controllable pace and allowed him to pursue a strong personal interest in patient education. His community health activities also served as a productive public relations tool for his practice.

An internist with a suburban practice in a metropolitan area wearied of his family-oriented practice. The patients with whom he most enjoyed working were business people. He also wanted to work fewer hours and be able to charge higher fees. Enlisting the aid of a marketing consultant, he relocated to a downtown high-rise corporate center and tailored his practice to corporate clients. He began by distributing a sleek brochure about the practice to his new corporate neighbors, then hosted an open house to introduce his practice. He adjusted his office hours to attract the new clientele: a couple of days a week, he opened the office at 6:00 a.m.; other days he kept late office hours. He offered appointments to high-level executives at their convenience. His new office is decorated in corporate style; the receptionist wears a business suit. For this physician, the new atmosphere and clientele make medical practice enjoyable again.

Another plastic surgeon resigned from a group practice to pursue his own interest—hand reconstruction. Though pleased with his location, he needed to attract new patients with the goal of adding more colleagues to what he hoped would become a recognized regional center for hand reconstructive surgery. With the assistance of a consultant, he is pursuing general media coverage of the hand rehabilitation field and of his own work, targeting populations for whom hand disabilities are a major handicap. His goals are long-term ones: to do something major with his life, and to leave something important behind.

Notes
1. *See* Healy, 22. Reprinted with permission of the *Wall Street Journal*, © Dow Jones & Company, Inc., 1989. All Rights Reserved.
2. Steptoe, 22.
3. Steptoe, 1.
4. Charles, 35.
5. Wells, 35.
6. Berrien, 336.
7. *See* Charles, 35.
8. *See* James, B1.
9. *See* "Disaffection of Doctors . . .," 12.
10. *See* Note 3.
11. *See* Barker, 3.

Part IV

AGGRESSIVE COMMUNICATION: PAID PROMOTION AND ADVERTISING

Newspaper, radio, and television advertising—forms of paid promotion—are considered aggressive forms of practice building in most parts of the United States. Of all the communication tools available, advertising is at the extreme end of the conservative-aggressive scale for a medical practice. The decision of how aggressive a marketing campaign to mount depends on the intensity of the competition in the area, local norms, and the effect an aggressive strategy may have on referral sources.

While advertising is one potential marketing tool, it is generally not recommended by consultants for most medical practices. There are, however, exceptions. Consultants say that for some specialties, such as plastic surgery and ophthalmology, in which word-of-mouth referrals are not a major source of new patients, advertising may be the only effective method of practice promotion.

In parts of the country where competition is keen, advertising has become standard operating procedure and is no longer considered taboo. Now that marketing efforts by physicians are reportedly sweeping across the country, advertising may follow suit. The vast majority of physicians, however, continue to avoid this form of promotion.

In general, public relations activities coupled with marketing research have been the most widely adopted promotion tactics. Nevertheless, there are instances when a more aggressive marketing strategy is indicated.

16 COMPONENTS OF A COMPREHENSIVE MARKETING STRATEGY

Muhammad Ali, the 1960s-1970s heavyweight boxing champion, is noted for his "I'm the greatest" claim. His colorful personality had as much to do with the extensive media coverage he received as his formidable ability as a fighter. While the public enjoyed Ali's antics, most people would look askance at a physician who would stoop to such self-aggrandizement. Aggressive marketing, however, need not imply self-promotion, and there is no question that some aggressive marketing strategies can enhance a medical practice and dramatically increase the fulfillment a physician receives from the long hours spent at work. At the same time, some of the more aggressive communication strategies perform a valuable public service by informing people of medical services available to them and educating members of the community about matters of health and medicine.

Developing a Marketing Plan

For such communication strategies to be effective, they must be carefully planned. That's why consultants insist on getting some facts first, before engaging in any promotional activities.

The first step is to follow the initial practice analysis process discussed in chapter 3:

Step 1: Assess the practice and factors impinging on it: the physicians' goals, the practice, the practice area, public perceptions about the practice, referral patterns.

Step 2: Identify community health care needs and compare services offered by the practice to those offered by its competitors.

Step 3: Define the patients and the patient populations that might ideally be served by the practice.

Once this information is gathered and analyzed, the planning process begins:

Step 4: Develop or fine-tune present services, if necessary, to meet the needs of target patients, current and potential, and to serve the physicians' personal and professional goals.

Step 5: Determine how to reach targeted patients, both current and potential, and how to increase referrals.

Step 6: Develop appropriate communication for those targeted.

The planning process is followed by implementing and evaluating communication strategies:

Step 7: Implement the communication plan.

Step 8: Evaluate by measuring satisfaction, cost effectiveness, and practice growth.

Step 9: Go back to steps 1 and 2 to update environmental factors and evolving patient needs.

Targeting

The most important part of marketing is targeting correctly, and, according to Julia Schopick, most physicians don't understand what this means or how to do it. Her advice: get to know whom you want to reach and who your ideal patients are. Target markets are those groups identified as the most promising ones for a practice. These potential patients can be segmented into groups differing in desires, resources, occupation, education, geographic location, attitudes, age, and so on. The examples below show some criteria commonly used to select market segments:

- Proximity—a general practitioner might want to attract patients of all ages within a two-mile or a ten-mile radius.
- Market concentration—a physician might decide to provide care to the elderly only or other special groups.
- Service specialization—a practice may decide to provide only one service, such as hernia repair, to all markets.
- Ability to pay—some practices exclude Medicaid patients.

The market segmentation process is illustrated on page 176.

Factors in Choosing Strategy

Marketing strategies for medical practices will vary, depending on a number of factors:

- Whether it is a new or established practice
- The stage in the life cycle of the practice

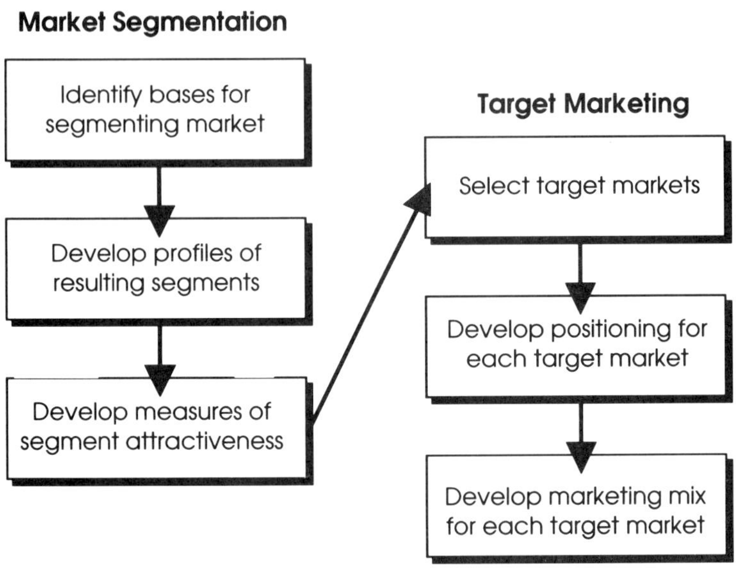

Source: Philip Kotler/Roberta N. Clarke. *Marketing for Health Care Organizations*, © 1987, p. 234. Reprinted by permission of Prentice Hall, Inc., Englewood Cliffs, New Jersey.

- The specialty
- Where the practice is located
- The goals of the practice
- Local norms

Whether a practice is new or established has been identified as an important variable in creating a marketing strategy.

In marketing a new practice, such objectives as creating an image, generating demand for the services offered, and creating community awareness are the focal points. In an established practice, the focus may be on improving the practice image, on communicating availability, or on attracting new patients.

Physicians' needs change with time, as do their practices. Consequently, practice life cycle stages have to be taken into consideration, according to Robert A. Fey, vice president for marketing and planning at a Baltimore hospital. As the table on page 178 indicates, marketing is important in the introduction and growth phases of a medical practice, a period of about twenty years.

The extent to which a medical specialty relies on referrals will also have an impact on planning a successful marketing strategy. For practices that rely to a large extent on referrals from current patients, a patient-oriented communication effort will be planned. For a medical practice that is largely consultative, a portion of the communication effort will be directed toward referring physicians. Medical specialties that rely on patient self-referrals will need to consider more aggressive communications, including direct-mail campaigns and advertising, particularly in competitive areas.

Local practice promotion norms should be given careful consideration. It may be perfectly acceptable to advertise on television in Las Vegas, but not in Kansas City, where physicians who do so may well risk losing referrals from angered, threatened, or offended colleagues. However, if a very specific and specialized service is to be offered in Kansas City, such as a hand reconstructive surgery, advertising may be the only way to attract a sufficient number of patients to the practice. Also, successful marketing strategies, though they may initially provoke disapproval, eventually gain acceptance.

Implementation

Promotion

Promotion involves communicating a physician's services to target markets and choosing appropriate vehicles to reach out to existing and potential patients.

LIFE CYCLE OF PHYSICIAN PRACTICE NEEDS

Stage	Age	Physician Needs	Response
Introduction	25–30	•Community placement •Startup capital •Marketing & financial support •Psychological support	•Act as a broker for retiring physician buyout •Low/guaranteed practice financing •Demographic analysis •Supply and demand analysis •Marketing support focus on patient awareness •HMO PPO introductions
Growth	30–45	•Networking •Marketing •Business management focus on revenue development •Office management •Access to capital	•Capital support for growth •Cross-sell physicians in direct market •Marketing support services focusing on penetration and expansion •Joint venture development •Satellite office analysis/ placement •Office management consulting •Computerizing office •Assistance with group practice formation
Maturity	45–60	•Convenience •Expense management/ more revenue per patient •Introduction of associates •Service specialization •Retirement planning	•Office management services •Hospital-based medical office building •Equipment leasing •Broker program to introduce new physicians to mature practice •Marketing support services focusing on segmentation strategies
Decline	60+	•Practice turnover plan •Flexible hours for pursuit of leisure •Stable income stream •Practice consolidation for "cash out"	•Practice valuation and buyout services •Part-time work through hospital •Teaching programs •Marketing services to minimize patient loss through transition

Source: Karen Super, "Services Should Be Linked to Practices' Life Cycles." *Modern Healthcare*, 17, © 1987. Reprinted by permission of Robert A. Fey, Greater Baltimore Medical Center.

A large number of promotional tools—from the generally acceptable preparation of patient education materials to the more controversial extreme, advertising— are currently in use by doctors. Whether a physician selects an informational newsletter to convey a well-established, professional practice or a direct-mail campaign to promote a new high-technology service, each communication leaves a perceived image with patients.

Promoting a medical practice can be costly and have negative repercussions. Those frequently listed are a loss of referral sources and a tarnished image for the medical profession. As a result, some practice management consultants and most physicians urge a cautious approach.

Never be more aggressive than you need to be, is common advice consultants give to doctors. "I've left promotion until last because that's exactly where it belongs," said Greg Korneluk. "Most doctors will never have to get to this point. Changes in product, price, or place will usually enable a physician to revive a flagging practice."[1]

Fees

While price can be a major component in a marketing strategy for products and is occasionally mentioned in conjunction with marketing of professional services, it has been found that fees are seldom a determining factor in choosing a physician. As a result, medical practice consultants ordinarily do not stress this marketing variable. Although fees are not an important determinant now, some practice management consultants view the growing trend toward higher deductibles and copayments by patients as a signal that doctor-shopping on the basis of fees may become significant and bears watching. The 1988 AMA poll showed cost of care to be a very important consideration in influencing choice of where to go for health care for 47 percent of respondents. Cost was of particular importance to senior citizens (60%) and to adults under thirty-five (42%). Fee strategies may become more important as patients are forced to pay a greater share of their medical costs.

Effective Marketing Need Not Be Complex

Korneluk relates that a California physician, confronted with a declining general internal medicine practice in a downtown location, wanted to increase his patient load. He determined through research that practically the only patients left in his area were elderly, and there was no immediate prospect for urban renewal that might bring younger patients into his practice. To take advantage of the situation or, in marketing parlance, to reposition the practice in the marketplace, he simply changed its name. By renaming it Geriatric Clinic, and placing a large sign outside, the physician again enjoyed a booming practice.

In any effective marketing plan, simple or complex, opportunities are identified and capitalized upon. That is the major purpose of any marketing plan. It is a blueprint for the future, one which facilitates logical decisions on how best to provide services, and how to allocate resources efficiently to accomplish goals, say consultants Leif Beck and Patricia Salmon.

Evaluation

After a communication strategy is implemented, it should be evaluated. Evaluation provides an assessment of the effectiveness of marketing efforts and the opportunity to fine-tune the marketing plan so that goals are attained as quickly and efficiently as possible. Professional marketing/public relations firms track marketing efforts and prepare progress reports based on goals and objectives set in the planning phase. For practices that do not employ outside firms, consultants recommend having one of the partners or an office manager follow up on marketing results through interviews, questionnaires, and tracking of patients and referrals.

A Caveat

The best-planned marketing strategy won't work if the practice is not patient-oriented, as the following case illustrates. The names of the entities have been changed to prevent identification.

MARKETING GONE AWRY? - A CASE.[2]

At the heart of the controversy over whether or not to market medical practices is the question of how much of a business orientation is necessary in medicine. Can a profit motive destroy a practice?

The most sophisticated marketing efforts can fail without an underlying genuine concern for the patient. That was the lesson learned by Med Serve, Inc., a chain of now boarded-up medical clinics in the Midwest, whose $100 forceps, $300 monitor attachments, stethoscopes, and other supplies were, in the end, heaped into dumpsters in the street.

Amid the realities of empty hospital beds and an abundance of doctors in the 1980s, medicine was changing. HMOs, PPOs, and cost-containment programs were making the health care industry increasingly complex and less lucrative for the solo practitioner. As these health care hybrids began to draw criticism, a business-oriented physician who, associates said, was more interested in profits than in patient care, made his move. The doctor, an internist with impeccable credentials from prestigious eastern medical schools, returned to his native Midwest after completing medical training. A private practice grew into Med Serve Professional Services, a chain of clinics serving Medicare patients, and a subsidiary, Park Avenue Private Physicians, Ltd., a slow-paced, high-tech practice that catered to the medical needs of rich patients, who were picked up and brought to the office in chauffeur-driven Mercedes limousines.

Doctors were recruited to the practice with the promise of financial security without the paperwork. They bought in at $75,000 (which soon rose to $150,000). These funds, according to contracts, would be used for promotional, advertising, and business development expenses incurred by Med Serve. It was a deal that appealed to physicians who were being squeezed financially and those who were overwhelmed by the new urgency to add marketing and business skills to what they preferred to concentrate on—clinical care. The clinics were staffed with board-certified physicians to assure quality care.

In 1985 the physician-entrepreneur teamed up with a savvy promoter known for taking fledgling companies public. "The prospectus was intoxicating—Madison Avenue medicine financed by Wall Street, Doc-in-the-Boxes that would proliferate like McDonald's and K-Marts." The prospectus boasted eleven clinics already in operation.

The idea appealed to investors. In its first two weeks as a publicly traded company, the stock shot up 438 percent on the over-the-counter market. By mid-1986, eight months after going public, it was trading at forty cents a share, a 700 percent increase. But the company would not complete a second year, despite heavy promotional efforts, which included the following:

- A slick magazine that dwelt on warning signs of various ailments and stressed the need for frequent medical exams

- $100 discount coupons good "toward a complete medical examination" (costing approximately $1,200)

- A program for Medicare patients that waived deductibles and copayments in exchange for a $10-per-visit fee

- A computer that at regular intervals scheduled appointments for patients and sent cards notifying a patient of the date and time of the appointment—without the patient's requesting it.

What went wrong? Essentially, the overpowering need to keep investors happy and the obsession to make money. To make the bottom line look better to investors, shady bookkeeping practices kept uncollectible fees on the books as accounts receivable. Questionable medical practices were encouraged, including excessive testing. Staff physicians were given financial incentives to order costly procedures during routine office visits, and their procedures were recorded on monthly "summary production reports."

The Med Serve culture and philosophy were profit-driven. The physician manual given to all doctors who joined the practice contained a reminder that insurance companies do not pay for "rule out" diagnoses. It predicted that Med Serve physicians would "accumulate a good deal of wealth." The section on relationships with patients offered the following advice: "You should explain, carefully, the necessity of routine Pap tests, sigmoidoscopies, and mammograms."

The practice of high-test, financially driven medicine soon led to an investigation by Medicare. A large payback to Medicare was negotiated, and no criminal charges were filed. As Med Serve began to unravel, it was discovered that as a result of leaving uncollectible fees in accounts receivable, presumably to please investors and to encourage further investing, income had been overstated by as much as $2.5 million.

The physician-entrepreneur resigned from the board and moved to another state. By October 1986 the clinics were shut, leaving a trail of lawsuits and a small amount of money, to be eaten up by legal fees. The numerous physicians employed lost their investments and their jobs.

Med Serve is a lesson in what can go wrong with bottom-line medicine.

"We have a long-standing reputation as poor businesspersons. And we should be proud that entrepreneurial success alone has rarely conferred high status in the medical profession," Dr. Philip Alper, a California physician, wrote in a letter to the *New England Journal of Medicine.*

When concern with the corporation's coffers replaces serving patients' health needs, the "business" can wither and die. In medicine, the best business advice seems to be Peters and Waterman's dictum to all businesses in *In Search of Excellence*: "Stick to the knitting." In medicine, that is the business of providing high-quality, patient-oriented health care.

Notes
1. Korneluk 1982a, 231.
2. *Source*: Mary Van de Kamp Nohl, "Stock Market Medicine." Reprinted by permission of *Milwaukee*, © 1987.

17 ADVERTISING: TOO MANY SIDE EFFECTS?

The photograph was a real eyecatcher: a brunette bombshell in a skimpy white bathing suit and silver spike heels standing next to a gleaming red sports car.

The caption was a real eyebrow raiser: "Automobile by Ferrari. Body by Forshan."

Forshan is Vincent R. Forshan, a California cosmetic surgeon who had never operated on the bombshell, a professional model. The photograph appeared in an eight-page fold-out magazine ad, which set Dr. Forshan back between $75,000 and $80,000.[1]

Although Dr. Forshan's advertisement is extreme and raises ethical questions, the increased exposure in the community from his foray into advertising made it worth the sizable expenditure, his ad agency claims. Apparently, it pays to advertise; Dr. Forshan, after his first success, is considering a second ad.

Pros and Cons of Advertising

For a medical practice, advertising is at the aggressive end of the promotional scale. As a marketing tool, it has been the focus of much controversy, and many questions have been raised by physicians and professional service marketers alike as to whether it is effective and appropriate for private medical practices.

After the Supreme Court removed prohibitions against advertising by professionals, many physicians jumped at the opportunity. *Television/Radio Age* reported that between 1977 and 1983, television advertising by doctors and dentists rose at an average annual rate of 48 percent, describing it as a growth rate just short of spectacular.

Despite a broader acceptance of marketing by physicians in the last few years, however, there is still much resistance to advertising. Local norms make it an acceptable practice in only small pockets of the country, including parts of Florida, California, and Nevada. Its relative advantage as a marketing tool for physicians is still in dispute, and only a small percentage of fee-for-service physicians advertise their practices.

Virtually every study has shown that physicians have fundamental reservations about advertising. Their fears center on the following issues:

- Concern that advertising will negatively influence perceptions of the profession, and further erode its image

- Unsuitablity of advertising as a means of communicating medical information to the consumer

- Conflict between medicine's focus on serving the needs of the people and the competitive nature of advertising

- Fear that advertising will result in antagonism by peers

- Doubts about the beneficial economic effects of advertising

- Relative unimportance of advertising in patients' selection or retention of a physician

- General suspicion of advertising by consumers and their consequent inattentiveness, unresponsiveness, or distrust

Physicians' skepticism about advertising seems to be well founded. Crane and Lynch's study showed that of the cues that consumers employ to select a physician, advertising ranked last. Consultants Donna Alexander and George Conomikes agree that some physicians will lose referrals if they advertise. "This could be deadly for a radiologist, delicate for an orthopedist who draws patients from physicians and the public, but no problem for a family practitioner who gets few referrals anyway."[2]

Studies have found that few doctors make use of advertising as a practice management tool. My own preliminary survey found that while six of ten advertising firms counseled physicians to advertise, only 12 percent of physicians were interested, suggesting that advertising firms attract fewer medical clients than public relations or practice-management consultants.

Is advertising, with all the controversy surrounding it, worth the price? A survey of 156 health care professionals who had previously advertised their practices found that advertising generated only 25 percent of new patients, compared with 63 percent generated by word-of-mouth referrals.[3] Perhaps with its high cost and questionable efficacy, advertising has little relative advantage compared with both marketing and public relations efforts, which can pack more punch at a lower cost.

Advocates of advertising by professionals argue that advertising of prices could, by engendering price competition, benefit the consumer by lowering professional fees. One problem with this argument is that only a small fraction of physicians' ads—6 percent—focus on dollar savings, and price is not yet an important variable in medical practice marketing. Also, while lower fees may result in an increase in net income, the increase is attributable to a higher patient volume, Festervand and Henthorne found. This implies that advertising makes it necessary to work longer hours to sustain the same income.

Consumer Attitudes Toward Advertising

Studies indicate that physicians should proceed with caution before they consider advertising. Hite and Bellizi report in the *Journal of Advertising Research* that consumers had favorable attitudes toward advertising by professionals (accountants, lawyers, and physicians) when all professionals were lumped together, with 80 percent of respondents reporting that they felt useful information could be provided through advertising. But when the three professional groups were considered separately, consumers were significantly less favorably disposed toward advertising by physicians. The study also found that consumers with a high degree of regard for the medical profession were least positive about physician advertising, which lends credence to physicians' fears that their image will be eroded by this marketing tool. The results suggest, the authors concluded, that physicians are viewed somewhat differently from the other professional groups by consumers, who appear to be more conservative about the business practices of physicians.

Although advertising is standard operating procedure for some medical specialties—like plastic surgery—and in some portions of the United States, most physicians have not embraced it. Overall, physicians are reluctant to advertise and are pessimistic about its effects.

One suggestion of a possible attitude change, however, arises from Folland's study of Pennsylvania physicians, only 3 percent of whom reported having used advertising. Over 47 percent of those polled said that they would increase their use of advertising if competition increased, and more than 15 percent said that they planned to increase their use of advertising during the coming year.

Medical Practices Need Different Approach

Because private medical practice really constitutes a public service, competitive advertising in the ordinary business sense seems inappropriate, implying as it does a desire to create sales revenues.

For physicians, imbued with a service rather than with a profit orientation, a different type of advertising may have to be developed, the purpose of which would be to inform rather than to sell services, Darling and Hacket suggest. The goal would be to provide objective information about the availability of service, special talents or expertise.

When to Advertise

The advice given by practice-management consultant, Michael Landry, regarding advertising by physicians best describes the consensus view of consultants: for a physician who knows how to market, advertising is not important. However, several medical marketing experts have found that although it is likely to meet with resistance, advertising does have some advantages in some instances and can be used successfully:

- When practices rely on patient self-referral
- When competition from alternative health care providers who advertise their services escalates
- When there is a glut in certain specialties
- In areas of the country where advertising is commonly used
- To inform patients of any change in a practice,

such as the association with another physician, a change of location or the addition of a new location, and new hours

- When a practice offers a highly specialized service

As the following case illustrates, some medical practices have found that ground-breaking advertising strategies can pay off, and that resistance may break down with time.

A MEDIA BLITZ SUCCEEDS—AFTER THE CONTROVERSY DIES DOWN.[4]

Medical advertising has been accepted as a marketing tool in parts of California, Nevada, and Florida. But when an extensive and innovative marketing campaign that relies heavily on advertising is instituted where such tactics are considered repugnant, physicians risk alienating their colleagues and thereby jeopardizing referral sources. They can also anticipate some fireworks.

Two New Jersey surgeons teamed up to insulate themselves from external forces that were destroying their practices. One was from an academic background and had published over thirty-five articles in prestigious journals. The other was a general surgeon who served as chief of staff at his local hospital. Both were fearful of what increased competition and decreased inpatient surgery would mean for their futures, and both wanted to remain in independent practice.

They looked for a high-volume operation that could be performed on an ambulatory basis, one that was not completely dependent on referrals. Hernia repair, the most common general surgical procedure performed in the United States, and a condition often self-diagnosed by patients, fit the bill. The Hernia Center opened in 1984.

After attending an AMA seminar on practice building and obtaining a $30,000 loan, the two doctors hired an advertising agency. The marketing strategy included a media blitz with the following elements:

- Advertising in fifteen New Jersey and New York newspapers
- Advertising on three metropolitan-area radio stations
- Providing a toll-free telephone number, 1-800-HERNIAS
- Discounting fees by 20 percent
- Offering one-price packages to unions, HMOs, and municipalities
- Performing surgery on Saturdays

The $120,000 campaign (20 percent of the doctors' gross income) brought patients from the entire metropolitan area—and the wrath of the local medical community.

The county medical society challenged the first ad for violating state regulations prohibiting the inclusion of sketches and drawings, and for not including the physicians' names. The name Hernia Center was misleading, claimed the society, because it implied a free-standing clinic, whereas the surgeons operated exclusively at area hospitals. The local medical community criticized the ads for their implication that the physicians had special expertise in hernia repair, a form of self-aggrandizement. Local physicians were also incensed by the fact that the surgeons had decreased their fees and induced anesthesiologists to do the same.

Neither the hostile letters from colleagues nor the establishment of an ad hoc hospital committee to investigate deterred the two surgeons. Gradually, the animosity evaporated. Business boomed, and the doctors report plans to franchise their marketing program and toll-free number to other physicians around the country.

In an interview, one of the physicians said: "Like it or not, this kind of marketing is the wave of the future. By promoting ourselves, we're able to maintain our independence and stay in private practice. I'd rather catch some flak for our 800-number than have to go work full time for an HMO."

Successful advertising strategies, though they defy local norms initially, are likely to be adopted by other physicians and to change those norms. According to the hernia surgeons, one of their original critics has asked them for advice on promoting his own practice.

AMA GUIDELINES ON ADVERTISING.[5]

There are no restrictions on advertising by physicians except those that can be specifically justified to protect the public from deceptive practices. A physician may publicize himself as a physician through any commercial, publicity or other form of public communication (including any newspaper, magazine, telephone directory, radio, television or other advertising) provided that the communication shall not be misleading because of the omission of necessary material information, shall not contain any false or misleading statement, or shall not otherwise operate to deceive.

The form of communication should be designed to communicate the information contained therein to the public in a direct, dignified and readily comprehensible manner. Aggressive, high pressure advertising and publicity may create unjustified medical expectations. Any advertisement or publicity, regardless of format or content, should be true and not misleading.

The communication may include:

a. educational background of the physician

b. the basis on which fees are determined (including charges for specific services)

c. available credit or other methods of payment, and

d. other information about the physician which a reasonable person might regard as relevant in determining whether to seek the physician's services.

Testimonials of patients, however, as to the physician's skill or the quality of his professional services should not be publicized. Statements relating to the quality of medical services are extremely difficult, if not impossible, to verify or measure by objective standards. Claims regarding experience, competence, and the quality of the physician's services may be made if they can be factually supported and if they do not imply that he has an exclusive and unique skill or remedy. A statement that a physician has cured or successfully treated a large number of cases involving a particular serious ailment may imply a certainty of result and create unjustified and misleading expectations in prospective patients.

Consistent with federal regulatory standards which apply to commercial advertising, a physician who is considering the placement of an advertisement or publicity release, whether in print, radio or television, should determine in advance that his communication or message is explicitly and implicitly truthful and not misleading.

These standards require the advertiser to have a reasonable basis for claims before they are used in advertising. The reasonable basis must be established by those facts known to the advertiser, and those which a reasonable, prudent advertiser should have discovered.

As used herein, references to a "physician" apply also to information relating to the physician's group, partners or associates. Any communication or message within the scope of this opinion should include the name of at least one physician responsible for its content.

Nothing in any opinion of the Judicial Council is intended or shall be construed to discourage or to limit advertising and representations which are not false or deceptive within the meaning of Section 5 of the Federal Trade Commission Act (II).

Notes
1. Shearer, 16. *Also see* Hughes, 1.
2. *See* Carrell, 22.
3. *See* "Experience Belies...," 1. Reprinted from *Marketing News*, 18, published by the American Marketing Association, © 1984, with permission.
4. *Source:* Mark Crane. "Does a Practice Need a Gimmick to Survive Today?" *Medical Economics*, Vol. 63, pp. 132-138. Reprinted by permission of Medical Economics, Inc., © 1986.
5. *Source:* 1984 Judicial Council Current Opinions. Reprinted by permission of the American Medical Association.

18 EFFECTIVE ADVERTISING STRATEGIES

In areas of the country where advertising is an accepted and expected part of promoting the medical practice, paid promotions—*Yellow Pages*, direct mail, newspaper and broadcast ads—can be effective practice-management communication tools. Effective advertising does three things:

- It targets a specific audience
- It offers some benefit to the reader/listener/viewer
- It calls the person to action

Reaching Your Audience

Medical practice ads should be directed toward the member of the family who exerts the greatest influence in the selection of health care services. Because the decision-making process is so variable, multiple messages and multiple appeals directed at both husband and wife should be developed, Festervand and Henthorne advise.

To reach today's busy and fragmented families, various media should be considered. Ads may have to be placed on television, radio, and in newspapers. Advertising agencies have information profiling the media habits of particular market segments and could assist with placing ads that will reach target audiences.

Repetition is crucial in advertising. A one-time newspaper ad or radio spot rarely brings a noteworthy response, and seeing or hearing an ad once or twice is usually not enough to get prospective patients to call for an appointment. In most cases, people must be exposed to an ad several times before they respond—by seeking more information about the practice or by making an appointment.

Since advertising relies on repeated exposures to get your message across, budget accordingly. Media planners rank advertising vehicles on the basis of cost per thousand persons reached, with the most cost-effective being those vehicles with the lowest cost.

Ins and Outs of Physician Advertising

In planning an advertising campaign, you must target the audience(s) and then determine how best and most economically to reach them. Questions to ask media sales representatives include:

- How many people will be exposed to the advertising campaign?

- How many repetitions will these people be exposed to?

These questions should be asked *before* the advertising medium is chosen.

Each advertisement must have some objective: to educate consumers, promote a service, or position the practice. Physician ads can present any of the following:

- Information about the practice
- Real-life situations
- Demonstration of a technique
- Solution to a problem

Advertising objectives may vary at different stages of a practice's life cycle and in different environments. A new medical practice or new service offered by an established practice will seek to inform potential users of availability. Marketing authority Philip Kotler says that in a competitive market, persuasive advertising, which aims at building preference, is most effective.[1]

Any claim made in an ad should be honest—and verifiable. A few psychiatric and chemical dependence clinics have begun running some questionable ads that guarantee satisfaction with service. Implicit in them is that these generally long-term problems can be cured with one stay at the facility. In fact, the ads guarantee only satisfaction with the physical facility in the first two days of the patient's stay. The guarantee does not extend to satisfaction with treatment, as the ads imply. It is best to refrain from such borderline advertising.

Factual Information Best

The survey of health care providers who had advertised found that the most effective advertising concentrated on the professionalism of the service, according to respondents. However, most consultants advise against this type of advertising, preferring emphasis on factual, verifiable information related to the practice, in accordance with AMA guidelines (see chapter 17). Perhaps one reason professionalism of service was used as the message, a claim difficult to verify, is that two thirds of the health care providers created their own ads without professional advice. That number was even higher for solo and group practitioners, 76 percent of whom created their own messages. Advertising professionals considered these ads to be amateurish, ineffectual, and a waste of money.

Advertising Tips

The name of the practice should be prominent in any advertisement. Too many newspaper ads designed by physicians give the practice name in small print at the bottom. Such advertisements promote the profession, not an individual practice, and are as likely to direct business to the competition as to the practice paying for the ad, according to Piesto and Redding.

These consultants also point out that if an unflattering picture is used in the ad, the image of professionalism is lost. "Expressionless photos make doctors look like the last people on earth patients would want to confront in an examining room," they caution.

In the survey of health care providers who had used advertising, the *Yellow Pages* were found to be the most effective advertising medium (by 37% of respondents), followed by newspapers (19%), direct mail (15%), television (9%), radio (5%), and magazines (4%).

Yellow Pages *Advertising*

Telephone book advertising is the most common form of paid promotion. The public needs telephone listings, and it would be a rare physician indeed who would not take advantage of this advertising vehicle.

Although marketing experts view *Yellow Pages* listings as a necessity, some caution that many physicians make the mistake of under- or overutilizing this medium. Advertising consultant Joyce Sherry relates that a cosmetic surgeon had himself listed in ten directories. When his patient base was analyzed, however, he found that most of his patients came from a much more restricted geographic area. At her suggestion, he placed one display ad in the large metropolitan directory, used column ads in the directory for the suburbs where many of his patients resided, and boldface (dark type) listings in the key neighborhood directory. This new strategy saved him money without adversely affecting the growth of his practice.

When your telephone directory renewal notice arrives, take the opportunity to investigate the various alternatives available for advertising in the white and yellow pages of your local directory.

Following are the available options for *Yellow Pages* ads:

- A plain listing in regular type
- A boldface listing
- A large boldface listing
- A column ad—a one- or two-inch high ad confined to a single column, often containing additional information about the practice
- A display ad, which can run from an eighth of a page on up.

Your listing(s) can appear in several locations: under the specialty (Guide of Physicians & Surgeons—Medical—MD), under the practice name, and/or alphabetically under each physician's name (Physicians & Surgeons—Medical—MD).

Recently, more practices have included details about location, hours, and specialty in their *Yellow Pages* listings. The key to effective *Yellow Pages* advertising is that the ad be simple, clear and professional. Use uniform typefaces and keep the artwork, if any, neat. You may include your logo or other symbol, a sketch of your building, or a map of your location.

Advertising consultants give these additional tips on using *Yellow Pages* listings most effectively:

List in your town or city directory, as well as in directories of nearby towns or suburbs from which you draw patients. Determine which directories are appropriate by analyzing your patients' addresses.

In a display ad, don't claim superior quality or make fee comparisons. However, you can state "reasonable fees" or "personal, caring attention to you and your family's health care needs." The majority of boxed display ads are two columns in width and include hours, location, the names of physicians in the practice and the specialty.

Whether or not you need a display ad depends on your referral base. The primary purpose of display ads is to induce new patients to call. If you are a specialist who operates chiefly by referral, a simple alphabetical listing is usually sufficient.

Explain in layman's terms what you do: Dr. John Doe, Dermatologist: skin diseases, skin cancer, skin surgery.

For more attention in the alphabetical listing, put your name in bold type or try a column ad, adding two extra lines under your name to provide your practice name and your hours.

The standard telephone book is joined by a variety of privately sponsored community or business directories. For a small fee, they will include your name and telephone number. Your local Chamber of Commerce can provide you with the names of these alternative phone directories.

Some consultants suggest that *Yellow Pages* listings may be most useful in a town of transients, where word-of-mouth referrals are not well established.

Criticism of Yellow Pages *Listings*

Even *Yellow Pages* advertising has come under attack—by physicians themselves. A study by Reade and Ratzan reported in the *New England Journal of Medicine* suggests that even this seemingly acceptable form of advertising may be misleading the public. Of 964 Hartford, Connecticut, physicians listed among sixty-one categories of specialists in their area *Yellow Pages* directory, 12 percent were found not to be board certified, prompting the authors to point out that specialty advertising may be misleading consumers. In the authors' view, only physicians who are board certified or trained in a specialty should represent themselves as specialists in the *Yellow Pages*. Apparently, this is a matter of some controversy, which remains unresolved.

Newspaper and Magazine Advertising

Print media advertising is not widely used by physicians, with local exceptions. In a survey of 150 newspapers in seventy-five U.S. cities, McDaniel and Smith found an average of only one physician advertisement per paper. The largest number of ads (38.5%) were placed to inform readers about some type of change in a physician's practice, with new location accounting for 16.4 percent.

The authors concluded that patient relations and publicity are a more important part of the promotion mix for physicians than print advertising.

A physician may want to confine print ads to the geographic area he or she serves. If so, a community or suburban paper may be preferable to a large urban paper. The cost will also be considerably lower, as newspaper rates are calculated on the basis of circulation numbers.

Keep newspaper and magazine ads simple, informational, and professional in appearance. Include your logo, name, address—and a map if your office is hard to find (see the sample advertisement on page 202).

LAKE MEDICAL CENTER
IS
ACCEPTING NEW PATIENTS

Internal Medicine
General Surgery

•8 Board Certified Physicians
•Complete Laboratory/X-ray Facilities
•Mammography Center

Call (614) 464-8864
Same-Day Appointments
and
Evening Hours

Combining the care and concern of a traditional
doctor's office with the convenience
of a modern medical center

All Major Health Plans Accepted
Medicare Assignment Accepted

Offices located at
331 E. Town Street, Columbus, Ohio

"Good Will" Advertising

Take advantage of the ads sold for school sports and graduation programs, religious organization bulletins, yearbooks, local community theater playbills, and fund-raisers for community organizations. Aiding these organizations presents an opportunity for advertising without repercussions.

Billboards

Billboards are rarely used by physicians, but they are available. Outdoor advertising specialists contract for use of a board for periods ranging from one month to a year or more. Firms can provide a list of the locations of all boards within their domain. Select a location—a busy intersection or a crossroad, for example—where you'll get the most attention from patients you want to attract.

Because billboards use huge print, your message should consist of a maximum of ten words. Ideally, your name, address, and phone number, perhaps accompanied by a photo or drawing, are all that will appear. A motorist cannot read more than that in passing.

Broadcast Advertising

Television and radio ads reach people in massive numbers. Per exposure, broadcast ads are relatively inexpensive. Because of the necessary repetitions, however, the total cost is high.

Station sales representatives are equipped with audience profiles, which indicate the characteristics of the audience and when your target audience is likely to be listening or watching. Ads can be staggered throughout the day to take advantage of lower rates during off-peak hours, and to reach a wider variety of listeners.

Radio and television advertising should be left to the professionals to produce.

Prepare for the Onslaught

Carefully planned and executed advertising campaigns may bring a flood of inquiries. To be prepared, a practice should develop a response packet prior to implementing its advertising campaign. Typically, the packet includes a cover letter, a brochure describing the practice, and a booklet or other material on any specific services being advertised.

In addition, secretaries and receptionists should know what medical problems the doctor(s) in the practice treat. One internist relates that in response to a direct-mail campaign, a call came in from a patient with hematuria. Never having heard the term before, the receptionist assumed it was not among the conditions treated by any of the doctors in the five-person internal medicine group, and referred the patient elsewhere. An alphabetical list of all diagnoses covered by a practice is a handy reference for any receptionist taking calls after an advertising campaign.

Gauging the Effectiveness of Advertising

In evaluating advertising, remember that many factors influence patient choice and behavior, that most people respond slowly to advertising, and that impact builds over time. It should also be noted that owing to the complexity of factors and sources of information that affect patients' choice of health care providers, evaluating advertising is a most difficult and often inconclusive task.

Measuring Impact

To determine whether a physician's advertising dollars are being well spent, measure an ad's impact by surveying target audiences. Ask the following questions: How many people read (heard, saw) the ad? Recognized it? Were able to recall the ad?

Impact on Mind

Advertising is intended to influence the minds of those it reaches, with the assumption that behavior will follow suit. Advertising tends to be most effective among those with the weakest opinions: it is more difficult to change minds already made up than to form opinions.

Different campaigns may be needed for different mind-sets. The goal may be to influence awareness, knowledge, opinions, expectations, acceptance, or preference. Pre- and post-campaign surveys are required to assess any such impact (see sample questionnaire below).

Impact on Behavior

Behavioral responses to physician advertising range from requesting information about a practice to considering information to making and keeping an appointment. Direct response to advertising can be measured by the number of requests for more information or appointments. If a thousand people call for information on an acupuncture facelift the day after an advertisement appears, there is a strong link between the ad and the calls. To determine exactly which ad was most effective in generating direct responses, consultants suggest altering the ad in some way.

Use a different name, box number, telephone number, or media outlet to determine which ad prompted the best response; or create different versions of an ad to assess whether one is more effective than another. Such devices as split runs of newspapers or split cable television commercials and randomized tests of different messages can also be used.

Always ask patients who call or come into the office where they obtained the information that prompted them to make (and keep) an appointment.

Financial Results

This is a measure of the net profit of an advertising campaign. Did income resulting from the campaign exceed its cost? What is the cost/benefit ratio?

Ask the questions below in a focus group, interview, or survey questionnaire to determine awareness, knowledge, opinions, expectations, acceptance, and preferences of target audiences. The answers to these questions suggest what factual information in the advertising has had an impact. To determine whether the advertising campaign was effective, ask the same questions pre- and post-campaign to assess any changes. Ideally, advertisers pretest messages to determine which one of several messages has the strongest behavioral impact.

SAMPLE QUESTIONNAIRE DETERMINING ADVERTISING'S IMPACT.[2]

1. *AWARENESS*: Increasing awareness depends upon the reach of an ad (the number of people or households exposed to the ad at least once during a specified time period), frequency (the number of times within the specified time period an average person or household is exposed to the message), and impact (the value of the exposure through a given medium). The first provider mentioned enjoys top-of-mind awareness.

If people know only one doctor in the category requested, that is the provider they are likely to choose for care when they need it, especially if they lack the time or motivation to consider alternatives. An advertising campaign should at least increase awareness.

These questions evaluate awareness:

When you think of an (ophthalmologist, cardiologist, etc.), which ones come to mind?

If you or someone in your family had (a particular problem or need), is there any provider in the community you could go to for help? (Yes or No)

If yes, are you aware of a particular provider who can help you with (the particular problem or need)?

2. *KNOWLEDGE*: Knowledge involves only facts about

or features of the provider or service. Knowledge may lead directly to preference, intention or behavior.

> What can you tell me about (Dr., service)?

If you seek specific information linking a service to a provider, you might ask:

> If you or a member of your family needed (a specific service), is there anywhere in the area you could go for it? If yes, where?

To differentiate competing options, ask:

> Do you happen to know where (a particular medical practice or service) is located? or, What services are offered by (a particular medical practice or service)?

> How are (the medical practice or service) and (a competing practice or service) the same? (This question can be repeated for each competing medical practice.)

3. *OPINIONS*: Subjective judgments determine whether a particular service or provider is deemed to be effective, reasonably priced, convenient, and so forth. Also, answers to many of these questions reveal what changes might be made in the services offered, what might be communicated to the public to promote opinion changes, and what sources of information people rely on to form opinions:

> What is your opinion of (particular physician or service)?

> How would you describe him/her/it if you were asked?

> How would you describe (competing practices B, C, D)?

How are they different?

Another option is to list such attributes as friendliness, effectiveness, price, cheerfulness, competence, and ask people to rate, on a scale of 1 to 5 or 1 to 10 (from strongly agree to strongly disagree), each provider in the area on these attributes. A physician who has a larger number of positive attributes has an advantage over competitors.

On a scale of 1 to 10, where 1 is cold and impersonal and 10 is friendly, how would you rate (a particular physician or service)?

or

In terms of warmth and friendliness, would you say that (provider) is much more caring, a little more caring, the same, a little less caring, or much less caring than (competing provider)?

Opinions may be further probed to determine what past experience or tangible features are responsible for them:

What is it about (physician or service) that makes him/her/it (competent, friendly, etc.) as you rated him/her/it?

How can you tell in advance how (competent, caring, helpful) (the provider) is?

4. *EXPECTATIONS*: Expectations about outcome of care go hand in hand with opinions about the provider's attributes. Where they exist, these expectations can be among the most powerful determinants of preference. The following questions can indicate people's expectations:

If you were choosing a doctor for (type of care), where do you think you would get the best results? or, If you required (type of care), which doctor do you think would provide the best results?

Questions may be more specific:

If you were pregnant, is there one obstetrician that you feel would be most likely to make sure you had a healthy baby?

Different expectations should be probed more deeply, with such questions as:

What is it about (physician's name) that makes you feel you will (have a healthy baby, breathe more easily, etc.) under his/her care?

What is it about (physician's name) that enables him/her to get such good results?

5. *ACCEPTANCE*: People may be aware of, know about, and have opinions and expectations regarding a number of physicians and services in the area. Acceptance indicates which ones they would actively consider should circumstances warrant. If patients' factual beliefs are in error or if their opinions can be changed, providers who are rejected have a basis for an advertising campaign. Providers who are considered can identify what features or opinions to reinforce.

If you (had a positive pregnancy test, found that you began wheezing every time you exercised, etc.), what sorts of things would you do?

If you or a member of your family were interested in (plastic surgery, maternity care, etc.), which providers would you consider?

Reasons for acceptance or rejection should be further probed:

Why is it that you would not consider (physician or service)?

6. *PREFERENCE*: Creating preference is the aim of most advertising efforts. Answers to these questions determine where a provider stands among available options and will signal people's intentions under certain circumstances:

Which would you say is the best (physician, service) in the area?

If you or someone in your family needed (a particular service), where would you go?

In an emergency, where would you go for care?

If your physician could not see you for a week, what would you do?

Comparison questions may also be used to gauge strength of preference:

Would you say (physician or service A) is much better, a little better, about equal, a little worse, or much worse compared to (physician or service B)?

More probing questions should also be asked:

What is the chief reason you would go to (physician or service)?

SAMPLE ADVERTISING CAMPAIGN EVALUATION.[3]

Reach	75% of target audience, 1 exposure minimum
Repetitions over 2 months	30%, 1 exposure; 25%, 2 exposures; 10%, 3 exposures; 10%, 4 or more exposures
Reading	15% read some; 13% read most or all
Recognition	25% recognized advertisement
Recall	19%, unaided recall; 31%, aided recall; 15%, correct identification of sponsor
Awareness	52% reported knowing that (physician or service) provides stress testing versus 35% pre-campaign
Knowledge	35% reported knowledge of physician A's office location versus 18% pre-campaign
Opinions	22% rated physician A as warm and caring versus 15% pre-campaign
Expectations	55% reported high confidence in good knee surgery results versus 18% pre-campaign
Acceptance	42% listed physician A as the one they would consider for maternity care versus 28% pre-campaign
Preference	18% listed physician A as the one they would consider for maternity care versus 10% pre-campaign
Utilization	New patients increased by 100 more

	than the month prior to the campaign (or same month last year)
Revenue	Additional revenue from 100 new patient visits: $6,500
Profit	$6,500 additional revenue less $3,000 cost of advertising campaign = $3,500

Notes

1. *See* Kotler 1988, 618-621.
2. *Source:* Robin MacStravic. "Evaluating Health Care Advertising." Reprinted from *Health Care Management Review*, Vol. 13, No. 3, pp. 45-57, with permission of Aspen Publishers, Inc., © Summer 1988.
3. *See* Note 2.

Part V

TOWARD REGAINING AUTONOMY: RECOMMENDATIONS FOR CONSULTANTS AND PHYSICIANS

19 RECOMMENDATIONS FOR MARKETING/ PUBLIC RELATIONS CONSULTANTS

Consultants must keep in mind that the practice of medicine is a service devoted to the health of patients. This service orientation is in keeping with the norms of the majority of physicians. Despite competitive pressures, violated norms may slow or even stop physicians from marketing their practices.

As health care becomes a market product, it must solve the classic dilemma of equity versus efficiency, says William Kissick. This is the challenge to health care marketers and to their fee-for-service physician clients: to keep financial priorities in perspective, and to restore the image of physicians as service-oriented, caring professionals.

With that in mind, the following recommendations are suggested:

Take a Long-range View

Physicians are confronting a credibility gap. Their income is at an all-time dollar high, averaging over $115,000, with 31 percent making $150,000 and above.

Yet in a poll reported in the *Wall Street Journal*, doctors said that concern, not cash, motivates them. That the public is not convinced of this is evident from press reports of public outcry against high physician incomes. Clearly, the public is questioning physician motivation, and weighing today's doctor against twenty-four centuries of respected healers.

Against this backdrop, consider a direct mailing that targets a well-heeled clientele, leaving little or no room in the appointment book for patients of lesser means. Should the white coat be replaced by a business suit to serve only high-paying customers?

Doctors today must consider the nagging question of short-term versus long-term gain. Will doctors again be able to muster enough public confidence to channel their own direction? Should the eroding image of the medical profession, which invites public distrust and government regulation of the profession, be of concern? Each physician should take a stand on these issues, and consider the future prospects for the medical profession.

Will advertising, a business technique for selling, improve the image? Probably not.

Will the "Doctor of the Year" award to a humanitarian physician who makes house calls when needed improve the image? A little, but it's only one example—and one which invites an unfavorable comparison with the majority of physicians.

Will a marketing plan to lure patients in for the doctor's benefit restore the reputation of American medicine? It could—if it is turned around to address benefits to patients.

The more closely practice enhancement is aligned with the promotion of health, and the more physicians display a caring demeanor and a service orientation, the lower the risk to the medical profession and the greater the long-term prospects for fee-for-service medicine.

Offer a Broad Range of Services and Fee Structures

Marketing medical practices is still an innovation in most of the United States, and the diffusion of innovation literature is relevant to medical practice consultants. Theorists define innovation as an idea perceived as new by an individual. Although marketing has been around for a long time, it is a new concept to many medical practitioners.

The role of consultants, referred to as change agents by diffusion theorists, is to link the client with the innovation and to make sure that the marketing strategy selected matches each client's needs and solves his or her problems. Everett M. Rogers, the well-known diffusion of innovation theorist, argues that commercial change agents, that is, those consultants who stand to make a profit, have low credibility.

That being the case, the client should be allowed to sample the innovation on a trial basis. If in that trial the suggested strategy can prove its efficacy, its success will speed the rate at which marketing strategies are adopted by fee-for-service physicians.

The implication is that in areas where marketing of medical practices is not widespread, the availability of a range of options and fee structures, from teaching physicians how to conduct their own marketing efforts based on hourly consulting fees to planning, implementing, and evaluating a marketing strategy based on a monthly retainer, may induce more physicians to seek consultants' advice.

Work Through Opinion Leaders

Physicians give greater credibility to colleagues, particularly opinion leaders, who have tried some innovation—for example, a direct-mail campaign to attract new patients, from which they have profited—than they do to consultants. Opinion leaders from within the ranks of practicing physicians who are willing to use new strategies should be sought out. Arnold Relman, editor of the *New England Journal of Medicine*, may be a highly regarded opinion leader in the field of medicine, but he is not a practicing fee-for-service physician who is concerned with practice stagnation. He is unlikely to try marketing strategies.

Opinion leadership is a local phenomenon. Lenox Hill Hospital will have opinion leaders different from those at New York University Medical Center, though both are in New York City. Opinion leaders at any institution can usually be quickly and easily identified by asking other physicians and hospital personnel whom they are likely to approach for information.

Opinion leaders should not be confused with mavericks. Just placing ads in a newspaper in the conservative Northeast doesn't make a physician an opinion leader. He may, in fact, be shunned by colleagues who consider his flamboyance demeaning to the profession.

Be Sensitive to Differences

Be aware of local norms and different medical specialties. Ignoring local norms may cost a doctor referrals from angry colleagues. Before suggesting a television advertising campaign, determine whether such an aggressive marketing strategy is locally acceptable, or whether the degree of competition in the area merits any drastic departure from locally accepted practice promotion standards.

If, on the other hand, a physician chooses to limit the practice to a specific procedure, such as dermabrasion, advertising may be the only way to attract a sufficient number of patients.

Practice Organization Variables

In devising a marketing strategy for medical practices, be aware that the organization of each practice and its referral flow are important determinants of communication messages and vehicles. Hill and Fannin's report in the *Journal of Professional Services Marketing* identified four types of professional service providers: individual practitioners, same-service partnerships, group associations, and multiservice integrated organizations. Each has its own characteristics. Whereas the individual practitioner's hallmark is personalized service, the group or integrated multiservice organization can provide greater convenience and a wider variety of services.

Of the four service types, Hill and Fannin found that a group practice is least likely to undertake any communication program, particularly advertising, to recruit clients because of its reliance on referrals from within the group. However, this conclusion is in direct contrast to the results of Sherman Folland's study of physicians' advertising behavior in which practice size was not found to be a strong determinant of advertising behavior.

Consensus Development Conferences

The National Institutes of Health use a novel approach to biotechnical innovation that may have adaptive value. To determine the consequences of new medical technologies, the NIH holds consensus development conferences with biomedical researchers, practicing physicians, consumers, and others to reach agreement on whether a given medical technology is safe and effective. After a panel has thoroughly discussed the technology in question, a consensus statement is written, which is then widely disseminated to physicians, the mass media, medical journals, and the public.

A panel of practicing physicians, patients, hospital personnel, and media representatives might prove useful in convincing practicing physicians that patients and the media need and want more information from their physicians about health-related subjects. The communication vehicles—a newsletter on how a new regulation will affect patients, a semiannual backgrounder for the press on medical issues—could be discussed.

Stress Relative Advantage

Successes achieved by innovators encourage others to experiment. The greater the benefit, the higher the probability that the innovation—a marketing/public relations plan—will be adopted by others. At the stage when early adopters of marketing strategies are prompting evaluation by their peers, communication media can play an important role by stimulating interest in the new approach, teaching the needed skills, and publicizing the results.[1] A relatively new medium that may spark physician interest is a floppy disk "brochure," which is reported to be a big hit and which could be sent to targeted physicians. Workshops at hospitals or clinics organized for the convenience of physicians may also be effective.

Along with outlining the advantages of enhanced communication and marketing/public relations programs, the skills needed by the physician to conduct a campaign should be addressed at workshops. Tornatzky et al. found that neither workshops nor information alone won converts to an effective new methodology, whereas instructive guidance achieved a modest rate of adoption by physicians.

Getting Your Message Across

Getting messages to busy doctors can be difficult. Howard Lewis, a professional relations counselor and medical editor, offers some tips for this purpose:

- Repeat messages often, emphasizing practical advice.

- Give priority to how-tos on patient relations.

- Work within established medical channels—hospitals and medical associations—or have your message conveyed through these channels.

- Write messages at the doctor's level of sophistication, and make every effort not to lump all physicians together, but to speak in terms of specialty.

As a method for gathering physician opinion, mail surveys employing state-of-the-art techniques have reportedly provided high response rates at low cost.

Notes
1. *See* Bandura, 142-171.

20 DOCTORS IN THE COMMUNICATION AGE

In a gloom and doom prediction that rattled a 1987 medical convention, nationally known health industry analyst Walter McClure said fee-for-service medicine would soon die, and that the doctor glut may force as many as 20 percent of physicians to leave medicine.[1] This is indeed a dire forecast, considering that AMA figures show that 76 percent of Americans obtain routine medical care from private physicians.

Beset as they are by public distrust, rising costs, increased competition and legislation, and criticism from within their own ranks, some physicians are questioning their choice of career. Others, perhaps more optimistically, are willing to undergo self-scrutiny and, in an effort to bring about desired change, are turning to other professionals for advice. They are learning that, above all, what patients want is a sensitive, responsive physician, one who is a skilled communicator. In this communication age, when presidents are judged as much by their ability to communicate as by their ability to govern, America's doctors are also expected to communicate effectively.

Some patients want more information than they have been receiving so that they can participate in medical decision making. Most want doctors to communicate a caring attitude. Medical societies want more doctors to play an active part in explaining both the capabilities and the limitations of medicine to patients, to the media, and to the public.

The burden is on doctors to get their message across—that they *do* care about patient well-being, that they *are* dedicated, ethical, and socially responsible professionals, and that they *do* attempt to rein in the cost of health care—but not at the expense of debasing the quality care each patient has come to expect. "What remains to be seen is whether doctors in this new climate will be able to maintain their influence and autonomy as advocates for their patients. To do that, I believe, they will have to rededicate themselves to the traditional ethics of the profession," says Arnold Relman.[2]

In this campaign to restore public trust, the principles of communication play a central role. By employing marketing and public relations strategies to position themselves as caring and expert professionals, physicians can gain the support of their communities and, at the same time, benefit their practices. There is no question that those marketing and public relations activities which promote health and enhance communication between physicians, their patients, and their communities will significantly improve the reputation of the medical profession.

Gloom and doom predictions are not, of course, new to the medical profession. Many physicians, particularly those recently retired or on the verge of retiring, allude to the 1940s and 1950s as the golden age of medicine, a period of rapid acceleration of medical science leading to the successful treatment of many disorders. But even during this period of hope and promise, problems that sound familiar today were plaguing physicians.

One of a series of articles appearing in June 1946 in the *Toledo Blade*, an Ohio newspaper, dealt with physicians opposed to a national health insurance system and accused the medical profession of defending its entrenched economic position. Other articles in the series unearthed unethical physician practices, attacked physicians for refusing to testify against colleagues in court, discussed variations in fees for specific procedures, and bemoaned the high cost of medical care and doctors' fees.[3]

That the concerns of physicians half a century ago have a certain déjà vu quality indicates that the cares of physicians today have a history. Though it is worth noting that some concerns continue to recycle through successive generations of doctors without resolution, there is a major difference between circumstances of a generation or two ago and what doctors are experiencing as we enter the 1990s.

In the 1940s and 1950s patients were clamoring for greater access to care. Doctors responded by instituting answering services, by providing telephone numbers at which they could be reached at night, by ensuring coverage while they vacationed. Patient needs were met, and patient satisfaction restored patient confidence. But perhaps the larger issues were postponed.

Answering services, coverage, and the like have become standard operating procedure. These solutions required no more than what comes naturally to most physicians—ingenuity—and yesterday's needs and wants became today's expectations. Today's needs, wants, and expectations may be more problematic, reflecting the increasing complexity of society. The solutions are far less clear cut.

Not only how, but whether physicians tackle the larger problems facing health and medicine will reflect their degree of dedication. Whether doctors retain their medical decision-making authority depends to a large extent on whether they take part in helping the public make informed choices. Doctors today must take a stand on the cost versus quality controversy and get their side of the story to the public. The public needs to know that, as cost-cutting efforts take hold, physicians have incentives to hold back treatments. In some HMOs, physicians' year-end salaries are higher if they minimize the use of consultants, hospitalization, and other services. And studies show that in the most highly regulated states, more patients die.[4] As quality of care suffers, so too does the reputation of the profession.

Physicians reportedly control 60 percent or more of health care costs through their decisions, and their services account for about 20 percent of national health care costs. They must explain to their communities that the pressures to hold back expenditures place a new strain on their obligations to provide quality care to patients. They must communicate the consequences of a preoccupation with cost that may already have resulted in less effective medical care in a country where high-quality care is considered a right. Under the fee-for-service system, when physicians provide interventions they deem necessary, the benefits profit both patient and physician.

The point is once more underlined: cogent communication is a must. For the public to understand today's issues and support medical community decisions, the physician must be an effective communicator.

As doctors continue to contend with such broad issues as ethical behavior, loss of autonomy, and economic survival, they must remember the fundamental prescription for the health of their profession: the patient comes first, and the doctor has to let the patient know it. Basically, patients' expectations are not difficult to define—or unreasonable. They have been clearly voiced. Patients want to know what's wrong, what the treatment will be, how long it will take, and what it will cost. They also want to know that their doctor cares about their health.

The business of medicine is health. Though a medical

practice has its business aspects and the current economic environment dictates a necessary self-interest on the part of doctors, it is possible to keep a business sense while avoiding a business stance.

In an eloquent *New England Journal of Medicine* essay, Philip Alper wrote that the commercialization of medicine is disquieting to physicians "perhaps because we instinctively sense that although there have always been some business aspects to medical practice, medicine, in the most fundamental sense, is not a business. There is also a point beyond which mixing medicine and business stops making sense."

Recognizing that medicine is a service makes good business sense. Mutually beneficial doctor-patient relationships and sound practice management go hand in hand: communication strategies are effective risk management techniques and among the best deterrents to malpractice suits. They are also among the most effective means of acquiring new patient referrals. But above all, gratifying doctor-patient relationships, always based on communication skills, are at the heart of a rewarding lifetime career.

The challenge to the medical profession is to regain its autonomy, to revive the art of medicine, and to make the most of a career in medicine while meeting the needs and wants of patients. The challenge to marketing, public relations, communication, and practice-management consultants is to encourage a communication process that balances the competitive needs of individual practices with the need to garner grassroots support critical to the survival of fee-for-service medicine.

Notes

1. *See* L. Page, 14.
2. Excerpted from material originally appearing in Arnold Relman, "The Changing Climate for Medical Practice," *The New England Journal of Medicine* Vol. 316, p. 333, © 1987.
3. *See* Schuler et al.
4. *See* Shortell and Hughes, 1100; Wall, 31.

REFERENCES

Allen, B., Wright, R., and Raho, L. 1985. "Physicians and Advertising." *Journal of Health Care Marketing* 5(4):39.

Alper, P. R. 1987. "Medical Practice in the Competitive Market." *New England Journal of Medicine* 316(6):337.

Altman, L.K. 1976. "Communicating With the Public: A Physician's Responsibility." *Bulletin of the American College of Physicians* 17(8):6.

Aluise, T. 1987 "Components of a Medical Practice Marketing Plan." *Journal of Health Care Marketing* 7(3):54.

American Medical Association (AMA) 1987. Personal communications. July-December.

Associated Press 1987. "Mean Income of Doctors Found to Rise 6.5%." *New York Times* 22 November, 43.

Astler, V. 1979. "The FMA Public Relations Program." *Journal of the Florida Medical Association* 66(5):566.

Astrachan, A. 1988. "Five Ways to Blow a Patient Interview." *Medical Economics* 65(12):116.

Bandura, A. 1986. *Social Foundations of Thought and Action: A Social Cognitive Theory.* Englewood Cliffs, N.J.: Prentice-Hall, 142-171.

Barker, T. 1987. "Marketing Can Be Useful Career Tool." *American Medical News* 30(2):3.

Barkin, K. 1985. "Emergency Physicians Mobilize For Safe Driving." *Insurance Review* 46(1):21.

Barson, D. C. 1984. "Professional Services Firms Represent Fertile Ground for Marketing Consultants." *Marketing News* 18(22):14.

"Basic Training Document: How You Look on TV May Be More Important Than What You Actually Say—Some Tips to Take with You to the Studio." 1985. *PR Reporter* 23(3).

Bays, K. 1986. "Changing Health Care Practices." *Vital Speeches* 52(6):183.

Beck, L. C., Anders, G. T., and Sweeney, D. R. 1985. "Staff Plays Role in Marketing Practice." *Pennsylvania Medicine* 88(9):36.

Beck, L. C. and Salmon, P. M. 1985. "A Checklist of Practice Marketing Ideas." *North Carolina Medical Journal* 46(6):345.

Beck, L. C. and Sweeney, D. R. 1985. "Marketing Medical Practice Begins Internally." *Pennsylvania Medicine* 88(5):32.

Berkowitz, E. N., Hillestad, S., and Effertz, P. 1982. "Marketing/Public Relations—A New Arena for Hospital Conflict." *Health Care Planning and Marketing* 1:1.

Berkowitz, E. N., Kerin, R. and Rudelius, W. 1986. "Marketing of Services." In *Marketing.* St. Louis: Times Mirror/Mosby College Publishing, 607-627.

Bernays, Edward L. 1987. Telephone interview.

Berrien, R. 1987. "What Future for Primary Care Medicine?" *New England Journal of Medicine* 316(6):334.

Blendon, R. J. and Altman, D. E. 1987. "Public Opinion and Health Care Costs." In Schramm, C.J., ed. *Health Care and Its Costs.* New York: W.W. Norton, 49-63.

Bockus, H. L. "The Doctor Image." 1974. *American Journal of Gastroenterology* 61(5):356.

Burton, J. 1986. "Medicine Goes Madison Ave." *California Business* 21:62.

Byerly, K.R. "Medicine and the News Media." 1968. *International Ophthalmology Clinics* 8(1):107.

"Can We Make a Better Doctor?" *NOVA*. December, 1988.

Carnegie, D. 1939. *Public Speaking.* New York: Association Press, 362.

Carrell, S. 1986. "Only Trick to Marketing Is to Do It Right, MDs Told." *American Medical News* 29(37):21.

Center for Economic Development (CED) 1987. *Reforming Health Care: A Market Prescription.* New York: CED.

Charles, S. 1987. Letter to the editor. *Wall Street Journal.* 20 May, 35.

Christensen, D. E. and Giese, T. D. 1988. "Assessment and Application of Patient Satisfaction Variables in Marketing a Psychiatric Practice." *Journal of Health Care Marketing* 8(3):47.

Cohodes, D. R. 1987. "The Loss of Innocence: Health Care Under Siege." In Schramm, C.J., ed. *Health Care and Its Costs.* New York: W.W. Norton, 64-104.

Cohodes, S. 1984. "How Patient Feedback Can Improve Your Practice." *Physician's Management* 24(3):253.

Cohn, V. 1986. "The Price of Malpractice: How the Crisis Harms the Relationship Between Doctors and Patients." *Washington Post*, 12 August, 12.

Coleman, J. S., Katz, E., and Menzel, H. 1966. *Medical Innovation: A Diffusion Study*. New York: Bobbs-Merrill.

Connor, Jean. 1988. Personal interview.

Corchado, A. 1989. "Folk Healers Stay Popular with Poor in Rural Southwest." *Wall Street Journal*, 4 January, 1.

Crane, F. G. and Lynch, J. E. 1988. "Consumer Selection of Physicians and Dentists: An Examination of Choice Criteria and Cue Usage." *Journal of Health Care Marketing* 8(3):16.

Crane, M. 1986. "Does a Practice Need a Gimmick to Survive Today?" *Medical Economics* 63(6):132.

Current Opinions of the Judicial Council. 1984. Chicago: American Medical Association.

Cutlip, S., Center, A., and Broom G. 1985. *Effective Public Relations*. New Jersey: Prentice Hall.

Darling, J. R. and Hacket, D. W. 1978. "The Advertising of Fees and Services: A Study of Contrasts Between, and Similarities Among, Professional Groups." *Journal of Advertising* 7(2):23.

Delbanco, T. 1988. "Can We Make a Better Doctor?" *NOVA*, December.

Diamant, A. 1988. "The Passion of Dr. Love," *Boston Magazine* 80(10):162.

"Disaffection of Doctors is Discouraging Medical Students and Potential Ones." 1987. *Wall Street Journal*, 10 April, 12.

Dolan, K. 1985. "Effective Marketing You Can Do Yourself." *Physician's Management* 25(2):344.

Dow, B. 1987. "Medical Group: Massachusetts Bad Place to Practice." *American Medical News* 30(42):10.

Driesman, M. 1989. Personal interview.

Droste, T. 1988. "Practice Enhancement: What MDs Want." *Hospitals* 64(4):44.

Duffy, J. 1967. "The Changing Image of the American Physician." *Journal of the American Medical Association* 200(1):30.

Duke, P. and Karr, A. R. 1987. "Dentists Step Up Services and Marketing as Competition Increases in Crowded Field." *Wall Street Journal*, 20 November, 31.

Ebert, R. 1987. "The Changing Role of the Physician." In C. J. Schramm, ed. *Health Care and Its Costs.* New York: W. W. Norton, 145-184.

Ehrlich, A. 1983. "Differences in Marketing a New Practice Versus Marketing an Established Practice." *Health Marketing Quarterly* 1(1):23.

Ehrlich, Mel. 1987. Personal interview.

Erhardt, J. 1985. "Let Your Patients Do Your PR Work." *Medical Economics* 62(2):80.

"Experience Belies Healthcare Professionals' Ad Fears." 1984. *Marketing News* 18(12):1.

Feingold, M. and Johnson, T. 1975. Letter to the editor.

New England Journal of Medicine 293(22):1155.

Ferretti, J. M. 1984. "Does a Doctor Who Markets Himself Have a Fool For a Consultant?" *Medical Economics* 61(24):101.

Festervand, T. A. and Henthorne, T. L. 1986. "Health Care Advertising Directed Toward the Family Decision Making Unit: Suggested Guidelines." *Journal of Professional Services Marketing* 2(1):123.

Fiorillo, J. 1984. "Direct Response Marketing Does Triple Duty." *Pharmaceutical Executive* 4(10):38.

Fischer, J. E. 1987. "Back to Hippocrates: The Physician's Role as Central to Medicine." *The Pharos* 50(1):36.

Folland, S. T. 1987. "Advertising by Physicians: Behaviors and Attitudes." *Medical Care* 25(4):311.

French, H. W. 1989. "Panel Acts to Increase Family Doctors." *New York Times* 5 March, 40.

Freshnock, L. 1984. *Physician and Public Attitudes on Health Care Issues.* Chicago: American Medical Association.

Friedman, H. and DiMatteo, R. 1982. *Interpersonal Issues in Health Care.* New York: Academic Press.

Gapan, P. 1985. "Consultant Offers Tips on Marketing For Physicians." *American Medical News* 28(6):3.

Gibson, J., Ivancevich, J. and Donnelly, J. 1985. *Organizations: Behavior, Structure, Process.* Texas: Business Publications, Inc., 532-535.

Glaser, R. J. 1987. "Publish (in the *Yellow Pages*)—Or Perish?" *The Pharos* 50(3):33.

Goleman, D. 1988. "Physicians May Bungle Key Part of Treatment: the Medical Interview." *New York Times*, 21 January, B10.

"Good PR Requires Research, Help of Pros." 1987. *American Medical News* 30(2):19.

"Good Relations Boost Practice Growth." 1986. *Modern Healthcare* 16(10):28.

Grace, J. 1980. "Bridging the Gap Between Medicine and the Media." *Canadian Medical Association Journal* 122(4):450.

Greenberg, N. 1987. "Build—And Protect—Your Practice for Eventual Sale." *American Medical News* 30(8):18.

Hall, J. B. 1983. "If the Doc's on TV, Maybe It's Because He Takes the PR Rx." *Wall Street Journal*, 23 August, 1.

Harlow, R. F. 1968. "Public Relations for the Doctor." *South Dakota Journal of Medicine* 21(3):64.

Harman, R. D. 1987. Letter to the editor. *Wall Street Journal* 20 May, 35.

Harvey, L. and Shubat, S. 1986. *AMA Surveys of Physician and Public Opinion on Health Care Issues.* Chicago: American Medical Association.

—— 1987. *AMA Surveys of Physician and Public Opinion on Health Care Issues.* Chicago: American Medical Association.

—— 1987. *AMA Surveys of Physician and Public Opinion on Health Care Issues.* Chicago: American Medical Association.

Hayen, D. O. 1985. "We Revived Our Practice Without

Resorting to Ads." *Medical Economics* 62(25):153.
Healey, W. 1986. "The Disaffected Doctor." *Wall Street Journal*, 9 July, 22.

Hecht, B. 1987. Personal interview.

Hershey, Nathan. 1982. *Hospital-Physician Relationships: Case Studies and Commentaries on Medical Staff Problems.* Rockville: Aspen, iii-xii.

Hicks, N. 1986. "Patients and Other Publics." *Public Relations Journal* 42(3):28.

Hilfiker, D. 1987. "The Profit Motive Harms Health Care." In Bach, J. S. ed. *Biomedical Ethics: Opposing Viewpoints.* St. Paul, MN: Greenhaven Press, 172-176.

Hill, C. J. and Fannin, W. R. 1986. "Professional Services Marketing Strategies in the 80s." *Journal of Professional Services Marketing* 2(1):11.

Hite, R. E. and Bellizi, J. A. 1986. "Consumers' Attitudes Toward Accountants, Lawyers and Physicians with Respect to Advertising Professional Services." *Journal of Advertising Research* 26(3):45.

Hoffman, B. 1982. "Do's and Dont's of Dealing with the Media." *Canadian Medical Association Journal* 126(4):408.

"How Physicians and Consumers View the Health Care System." 1984. *Medical Marketing and Media* 19(4):11.

Hughes, K. 1988. "Body Not Perfect? Nose Too Large? Chest Too Small?" *Wall Street Journal*, 2 August, 1.

James, F. E. 1987. "Medical Expenses Resist Controls and Keep Going One Way: Higher." *Wall Street Journal*, 29 September, 41.

James, F. E. 1989. "Are Ad Campaigns a Cure for Ailing Medical Schools?" *Wall Street Journal* 25 April, B1.

Jensen, J. 1986. "Women Pick the Providers who Treat Their Illnesses, Those of Their Children." *Modern Healthcare* 16(10):66.

—— 1987a. "40% of Physicians Said They Would Increase Admissions to Hospitals That Provide Management and Marketing Help." *Modern Healthcare* 17(14):130.

—— 1987b. "Most Physicians Believe Patients Obtain Healthcare Information from Mass Media." *Modern Healthcare* 17(19):110 .

Jensen, J. and Miklovid, N. 1986. "Consumers Cite Physicians' Interest as Most Important Factor in Selection." *Modern Healthcare* 16(2):48.

"Joint Ventures Multiply in Health Care Marketing." 1985. *Marketing News* 19(24):28.

Judd, W. H. 1967. "Can the Best Be Better?" *The Journal of the Kentucky Medical Association* 65(3):271.

—— 1969. "The Physician's Responsibility as a Citizen." *Nebraska Medical Journal* 54(12):771.

Kaplan, A. 1985. "Using the Components of the Marketing Mix To Market Emergency Services." In W. Winston, ed. *Marketing Ambulatory Care Services.* New York: Hawthorne Press, 53-62.

Kaplan, E. 1988. "Marketing/Public Relations in the Management of the Fee-for-Service Medical Practice." M.S. Thesis, Boston University, College of Communication.

Kiely, T. 1987. "Philip Johnston: On the Modern Challenges to Massachusetts Physicians." *Massachusetts Medicine* 2(4):11.

Kirkland, D. 1988. "How To Get Your Name Into The News." *American Medical News* 31(3):13.

Kissick, W. L. 1986. "Health Care in the '80's: Changes, Consequences and Choices." *Vital Speeches* 52(7):213.

Kleinfield, N. R. 1986. "A Squeeze on Doctor's Profits: Even the Group Practices Have Been Hurt By Medicare Rules, High Costs and New Competition." *New York Times.* 2 June, F1.

Knox, R. 1988. "Mass. Doctors on Increase Since '76, Study Says." *Boston Globe* 18 December, 33.

Korcok, M. 1982. "Marketing Your Services—A Matter of Patient PR." *Canadian Medical Association Journal* 126(3):301.

Korneluk, G. N. 1982a. "What Marketing Really Means for a Doctor." *Modern Economics* 59(4):225.

—— 1982b. "Marketing Myths, Mystiques and Misconceptions." *Canadian Doctor* 48(8):27.

Kotler, P. 1988. *Marketing Management.* Englewood Cliffs, N.J.: Prentice-Hall.

Kotler, P. and Clarke, R. 1987. *Marketing for Health Care Organizations.* Englewood Cliffs, N.J.: Prentice-Hall.

Kotler, P. and Mindak, W. 1978. "Marketing and Public Relations." *Journal of Marketing* 42:13.

Kurtzman, J. 1988. "Prospects." *New York Times*, 27 November, 1.

Kviz, F. J. 1984. "Attitudes Toward Physician Advertising Among Rural Consumers." *Medical Care* 22(4):300.

"Labor Letter." 1987. *Wall Street Journal*, 28 July, 1.

Leaverton, L. E. 1968. "Too Much About Public Relations?" *Journal of the Iowa Medical Society* 58(5):523.

Leebov, W. and Goldsmith, M. 1984. "How to Create a More Consumer-Oriented Work Force." *Personnel Administrator* 29(10):99.

Lehman, B. A. 1989. "Who Should Call the Shots?" *Boston Globe*, 6 March, 29.

Lesly, P. 1983. *Lesly's Public Relations Handbook*. Engelwood Cliffs, N.J.: Prentice-Hall.

Levine, E. 1987. "Physician Broadcasters." *Massachusetts Medicine* 2(4):38.

Lewis, H. R. 1977. "How to Get Your Message Across to Doctors." *Public Relations Quarterly* 22(4):20.

Lipkin, M. 1987. "The Medical Interview and Related Skills." In W. Branch, ed. *Office Practice of Medicine*. Philadelphia: W. B. Saunders, 1287-1306.

—— 1989. Telephone interview.

Long, J. 1984. "Look Who's Helping Build Practices Now." *Medical Economics* 61(25):75.

"Looking Back at Floppy Ads, Men's Hair Coloring and More." 1987. *Wall Street Journal*, 31 December, 9.

Lowe, C. U. 1980. "The Consensus Development Program: Technology Assessment at the National Institute of Health." *British Medical Journal* 280(6231):1583.

Lutz, S. 1987. "Marketing, Public Relations are Keys to Outpatient Surgery Business." *Modern Healthcare* 17(4):96.

MacStravic, R. S. 1987. "Manageable Evidence in Medical Care Marketing." *Journal of Health Care Marketing* 7(4):52.

—— 1988. "Evaluating Health Care Advertising." *Health Care Management Review* 13(3):45.

Mangold, W. G., Berl, R., Pol, L. and Abercrombie, C. L. 1987. "An Analysis of Consumer Reliance on Personal and Nonpersonal Sources of Professional Service Information." *Journal of Professional Services Marketing* 2(3):9.

"Marketing." 1987. *Wall Street Journal*, 29 October, 35.

Massachusetts Medical Society (MMS). 1987. Personal communication, July-September.

Mathieu, P. L. 1975. "The Doctor as a Revolutionary: The Next Twenty Five Years." *Rhode Island Medical Journal* 58(4):175.

McCullough, V. E. 1987. "Writing a Book a Good Way to Enhance MD's Image." *American Medical News* 30(24):16.

McDaniel, S., Smith, L., and Smith, K. 1986. "The Status of Physician Advertising." *Journal of Professional Services Marketing* 2(1):131.

"MD-Patient Communications Stressed." 1987. *American Medical News* 30(37):25.

Mercer Meidinger Hansen. 1987. "What Medicine Will Look Like in the Year 2000." *The Bulletin* 144, June.

Miller, J. A. and Waller, R. 1979. "Health Care Advertising: Consumer vs. Physician Attitudes." *Journal of Advertising* 8(4):20.

Moore, G. 1988. "Can We Make a Better Doctor?" *NOVA*, December.

Morgan, T. W. 1980. "Communications, Credibility and

Public Image." *Ohio State Medical Journal* 76(2):78.

Morreim, E. H. 1987. "Physicians Face New Ethical Binds." *Wall Street Journal*, 24 September, 26.

Nohl, M. V. 1987. "Stock Market Medicine." *Milwaukee*, July, 34.

Norman, J. 1988. "Would It Pay You to Hire a Management Consultant?" *Medical Economics* 65(11):50.

Ohio State Medical Association Department of Communications and Physician Marketing. 1987a. "Packaging Your Practice." *Ohio Medicine* 83(11):769.

—— 1987b. "Treating Your Practice-I." *Ohio Medicine* 83(12):867.

—— 1988a. "Treating Your Practice-II." *Ohio Medicine* 84(1):49.

—— 1988b. "Treating Your Practice-III." *Ohio Medicine* 84(2):145.

—— 1988c. "Getting Professional Help." *Ohio Medicine* 84(3):206.

"OSMA Public Opinion Survey Assesses Attitudes on Issues in Medicine." 1983. *Journal of the Oklahoma State Medical Association* 76(1):13.

Okrent, D. 1987. "You and the Doctor: Striving for a Better Relationship." *New York Times Magazine*. 29 March, 18.

Owens, A. 1985. "Doctor's Earnings: The Year of the Big Surprise." *Medical Economics* 62(18):194.

—— 1986. "1995: Who Will Be Your Patients?" *Medical Economics* 63(7):35.

Page, I. H. 1970. "Science Writers, Physicians and the Public—Ménage à Trois." *Annals of Internal Medicine* 73(4):641.

Page, J. 1987. "A Prescription for Medicine." *Annals of Emergency Medicine* 16(1):120.

Page, L. 1987. "Finances Will Put Some MDs, Hospitals Out of Business." *American Medical News* 30(20):14.

Pear, R. 1987. "Physicians Contend Systems of Payment Have Eroded Status." *New York Times*, 26 December, 1.

Peters, T. and Waterman, R. 1982. *In Search of Excellence.* New York: Warner Books.

"Physicians Must Know Their Patients, Competitors, Service Areas to Effectively Market Their Practices." 1986. *Marketing News* 20:15.

"Physician Marketing Budgets to Grow in '88." 1988. *Hospitals* 62(2):32.

Piesto, G. and Redding, W. 1987. "Marketing: How To Do It Effectively and Quietly." *Physician's Management* 27(10):111.

"Preparing for a TV Appearance." 1979. *PR Reporter* 17(7).

"Public Thinks Clergy, Doctors, Public School Staffs Contribute Most to Society." 1981. *Gallup Report* 193:15.

Reade, J. M. and Ratzan, R. M. 1987. "Yellow Professionalism: Advertising By Physicians in the *Yellow Pages*." *New England Journal of Medicine* 316:1315.

Relman, A. S. 1987. "The Changing Climate for Medical Practice." *New England Journal of Medicine* 316(6):333.

Relman, A. S. and Reinhardt, U. 1986. "Medicine As Business: Are Doctors Entrepreneurs?" *Science* 233(4768):1032.

Renn, S. C. 1987. "The Structure and Financing of the Health Care Delivery System in the 1980's." In C. J. Schramm, ed. *Health Care and Its Costs.* New York: W. W. Norton, 8-48.

Ricardo-Campbell, R. 1986. "Economics and Health." *Vital Speeches* 52(11):345.

Roe, B. B. 1978. "Professional Advertising: Ground Rules for Ethical Relations With the Communications Media." *The Annals of Thoracic Surgery* 26(1):1.

Rogers, D. E. 1988. *Clinical Education and the Doctor of Tomorrow.* New York: New York Academy of Medicine, November.

Rogers, E.M. 1962. *Diffusion of Innovations.* New York: Free Press of Glencoe.

—— 1983. *Diffusion of Innovations.* New York: The Free Press.

Rogers, E.M. and Shoemaker, F. F. 1971. *Communications of Innovations: A Cross-Cultural Approach.* New York: The Free Press.

Rosenthal, S. B. 1989. "The Myths of Malpractice." *Boston Globe,* 17 January, 15.

Ross, C. K. et al. 1987. "The Role of Expectations in Patient Satisfaction With Medical Care."*Journal of Health Care Marketing* 7(4):16.

Rubin, D. M. and Hendy, V. 1977. "Swine Influenza and the News Media." *Annals of Internal Medicine* 87(6):769.

Ruffenach, G. 1988. "Big Changes Proposed for Doctors' Fees." *Wall Street Journal*, 9 September, 23.

—— 1988. "Health Costs." *Wall Street Journal*, 11 October, B1.

"Rx: Public Relations." 1985. *Public Relations Journal* 41(4):10.

Sammons, J. 1987. Letter to the editor. *Wall Street Journal*, 20 May, 35.

Sandson, J. I. 1987. "How Many Physicians Are Enough?" *Boston University Medical Center Centerscope* 18(1):2.

Schopick, J. E. 1987a. "Public Relations Brings Visibility, Credibility—For Free." *American Medical News* 30(14):15.

—— 1987b. "Dispelling Five Myths About Public Relations." *American Medical News* 30(28):14.

—— 1987c. "Avoid Common Mistakes in Your Public Relations Efforts." *American Medical News* 30(39):15.

Schuler, E., Mowitz, R. and Mayer, A. 1952. *Medical Public Relations*. Detroit: Academy of Medicine of Toledo and Lucas County, Ohio.

Schwartz, H. 1986. "The Veterinarian Ethic." *Wall Street Journal*, 9 July, 22.

Selden, T. 1966. "Office Hints." *Anesthesia and Analgesia* 45(1):133.

Shahady, E. J. 1987. "Marketing Your Practice—How It Can Be Ethical." *Consultant* 27(3):90.

Shapiro, R. Y. and Young, J.T. 1986. "The Polls: Medical

Care in the U.S." *Public Opinion Quarterly* 50(3):418.
Shearer, L. 1988. "A Doctor Who Advertises." *Parade*, 24 July, 16.

Sherry, J. 1987. "Practice Promotion Can Keep, Boost Patient Base." *American Medical News* 30(13):15.

Shimp, T. and Preston, I. 1981. "Deceptive and Nondeceptive Consequences of Evaluative Advertising." *Journal of Marketing*, 45:22.

Shochet, B. R. 1986. "As Others See Us." *Maryland Medical Journal* 35(12):999.

Shortell, S. and Hughes, E. F. 1988. "The Effects of Regulation, Competition, and Ownership On Mortality Rates Among Hospital Inpatients." *New England Journal of Medicine* 318(17):1100.

Shosteck, H. and Fairweather, W. R. 1979. "Physician Response Rates to Mail and Personal Interview Surveys." *Public Opinion Quarterly* 43(2):206.

Soutter, L. 1970. "The Physician and the Community." *Bulletin of the New York Academy of Medicine* 46(7):489.

Stankaitis, J. A. 1987. "The Physician-Patient Relationship in Interesting Times." *New York State Journal of Medicine* 87(10):553.

Starfield, B. et al. 1981. "The Influence of Patient-Practitioner Agreement on Outcome of Care." *American Journal of Public Health* 71(2):127.

Starr, P. 1982. *The Social Transformation of American Medicine*. New York: Basic Books.

Steptoe, S. 1987. "Hassles and Red Tape Destroy Joy of the Job for Many Physicians." *Wall Street Journal*, 10 April, 1.

Super, K. E. 1986a. "Good Relations Boost Practice Growth."*Modern Healthcare* 16(10):28.

—— 1986b. "Memorial Hospital Emphasizes Guest Relations to Attract Patients." *Modern Healthcare* 16(18):42.

—— 1987. "Services Should Be Linked to Practices' Life Cycles." *Modern Healthcare* 17(8):57.

Tellem, S. 1987. Personal communication.

"Too Many Doctors." 1988. *Wall Street Journal*, 6 December, 1.

Tornatzky, L. G. et al. 1980. *Innovation and Social Process: A National Experiment in Implementing Social Technology*. New York: Pergamon Press.

Tursi, F. M. 1984. "Our Walk-In Clinic Beat Hospitals to the Punch." *Medical Economics* 61(26):89.

Van Doren, D. C. and Smith, L. W. 1987. "Physician Marketing in the Restructured Medical Services Field." *Journal of Health Care Marketing* 7(3):7.

Wall, W. 1988. "Cost Cuts Are Seen Hurting Health Care." *Wall Street Journal*, 28 April, 31.

Wallace, C. 1987. "Treatment Guarantees to Proliferate Despite Claims That Ads Are Misleading." *Modern Healthcare* 17(15):40.

Wallen, E. 1985. "Competition Prods Physicians Into Medical Marketing." *Physicians Financial News* 3(7):1.

—— 1987. "Concept of Medical Marketing Gets Growing Acceptance From Doctors." *Physicians Financial News* 5(8):B1.

Weddon, W. 1981. "Amway Founder Tells Physicians to Stop Apologizing." *Michigan Medicine* 80(29):562.

Wells, R. 1987. Letter to the editor. *Wall Street Journal*, 20 May, 35.

Welton, D. G. 1967. "Surviving in Today's Society." *North Carolina Medical Journal* 28(4):152.

White, E. E. 1979. "M.D.'s Image Depends 5% on Media, 95% on Doctor/Patient Relationship." *Michigan Medicine* 78(17):312.

Wright, R. A. and Allen, B. H. 1983. "Marketing and Medicine: Why Advertising is Not an Issue." *Journal of the American Medical Association* 250(1):47.

INDEX

American College of Physicians for "Science Writers, Physicians and the Public—Menage a Trois" by I. Page, *Annals of Internal Medicine* Vol. 73 p. 641, © 1970.
American Marketing Association for "Physicians Must Know Their Patients, Competitors, Service Areas to Effectively Market Their Practices," *Marketing News* Vol. 20 p. 15, © 1986; "Experience Belies Healthcare Professionals' Ad Fears ," *Marketing News* Vol. 18 p. 1, © 1984; "Manageable Evidence in Medical Care Marketing by R. MacStravic, *Journal of Health Care Marketing* Vol. 7 p. 52, © 1987; and "Consumer Selection of Physicians and Dentists: An Examination of Choice Criteria and Cue Usage," *Journal of Health Care Marketing* Vol. 8 p. 16, © 1988.
American Medical Association for *AMA Guidelines on Advertising* , 1984; AMA *Surveys of Physician and Public Opinion on Health Care Issues* by L. Harvey and S. Shubat, © 1986, 1987.
American Medical News for "Dispelling Five Myths About Public Relations " Vol. 30 No. 28 p. 14, © 1987; "Avoid Common Mistakes in Your Public Relations Effort " Vol. 30 No. 39 p. 15, © 1987; "Public Relations Brings Visibility, Credibility—For Free " Vol. 30 No. 14 p. 15, © 1987, all by J. Schopick; "Marketing can be Useful Career Tool" by T. Barker, Vol. 30 No. 2 p. 3, © 1987; "Only Trick to Marketing is to Do It Right, MD's Told" by S. Carrell, Vol. 29 No. 37 p. 21, © 1986; "Practice Promotion Can Keep, Boost Patient Base" by J. Sherry, Vol. 30 No. 13 p. 15, © 1987; "How to Get Your Name Into the News" by D. Kirkland, Vol. 31 No. 3 p. 13, © 1988; and "Finances Will Put Some MD's, Hospitals Out of Business" by L. Page, Vol. 30 No. 20 p. 14, © 1987.
Aspen Publishers for "Evaluating Health Care Advertising" by R. MacStravic, *Health Care Management Review* Vol. 13, p. 45, © 1988; and *Hospital Physican Relationships: Case Studies and Commentaries on Medical Staff Problems* by N. Hershey, © 1982.
Associated Press for "Mean Income of Doctors Found to Rise 6.5%~" (*New York Times* November 22, 1987) © 1987.
The Canadian Medical Association for "Marketing Your Services - A Matter of Patient PR" by M. Korcok, *Canadian Medical Association Journal* Vol. 126 p. 301, © 1982; "Do's and Don'ts of Dealing with the Media" by H. Hoffman, *Canadian Medical Association Journal* Vol. 126 p. 408, © 1982; and "Bridging the Gap Between Medicine and the Media" by J. Grace, *Canadian Medical Association Journal* Vol. 122 p. 450, © 1980.
City News Publishing Co. for "Health Care in the '80*s: Changes, Consequences and Choices"* by W. Kissick, *Vital Speeches* Vol. 52 p. 213, © 1986.

Crane Communications for "Services Should be Linked to Practices' Life Cycles" by K. Super, *Modern Healthcare* Vol. 17 p. 56, © 1987; "40% of Physicians Said They Would Increase Admissions to Hospitals that Provide Management and Marketing Help" by J. Jensen, *Modern Healthcare* Vol. 17 p. 130, © 1987; and "Most Physicians Believe Patients Obtain Healthcare Information from Mass Media" by J. Jensen, *Modern Healthcare* Vol. 17 p. 110, © 1987.

Dow Jones & Company, Inc . for "Dispirited Doctors : Hassles and Red Tape Destroy Joy of the Job for Many Physicians " by S. Steptoe, (*Wall St. Journal* April 10, 1987), © 1987; "Big Changes Proposed for Doctors' Fees " by R. Ruffenach (*Wall St. Journal* September 9, 1988), © 1988, and "The Disaffected Doctor (*Wall St. Journal* July 9, 1986), © 1986.

Harcourt Brace Jovanovich, Inc. for "How Patient Feedback Can Improve Your Practice" by S. Cohodes, *Physician's Management* Vol. 24 p. 253, © 1984.

Journal of the Florida Medical Association for "The FMA Public Relations Program" by V. Astler, Vol. 66 p. 566, © 1979.

J. P. Lippincott Co. for "Advertising by Physicians: Behaviors and Attitudes" by S. Folland, *Medical Care* Vol. 25 p. 311, 1987.

Little, Brown & Co. for "Medicine and the News Media " by K. Byerly, *International Ophthalmology Clinics* Vol. 8 p. 107, © 1968.

Maryland Medical Journal for "As Others See Us" by B. Shochet, Vol. 35 p. 999, © 1986.

Medical Economics for "Doctor's Earnings: The Year of the Big Surprise" by A. Owens, Vol. 62 p. 194, © 1985; "Does a Practice Need a Gimmick to Survive Today?" by M. Crane, Vol. 63 p. 132, 1986; "What Marketing Really Means for a Doctor" by G. Korneluk, Vol. 59 p. 225, 1982; "Let Your Patients Do Your PR Work" by J. Erhardt, Vol. 62 p. 80, © 1985; and "Five Ways to Blow a Patient Interview" by A. Astrachan, Vol. 65 p. 116, © 1988.

Michigan State Medical Society for "Amway Founder Tells Physicians to Stop Apologizing" by W. Weddon, *Michigan Medicine* Vol. 80 p. 562, © 1981.

Milwaukee Magazine, Inc. for "Stock Market Medicine" by M. Nohl, July, 1987, p. 34, © 1987.

C.V. Mosby Co. for "Marketing of Services" by E.N. Berkowitz, R. Kerin and W. Rudelius, in *Marketing* , pp. 607-627, © 1986.

New York State Journal of Medicine for "The Physician-Patient Relationship in Interesting Times" by J. Stankaitis, Vol. 87 p. 533, © 1987.

The *New England Journal of Medicine* for "The Changing Climate for Medical Practice" by A. Relman, Vol. 16 p. 333, © 1987.
The New York Times for "Physicians May Bungle Key Part of Treatment: The Medical Interview " by Daniel Goleman (January 21, 1988), © 1988; and "Physicians Contend Systems of Payment Have Eroded Status " by Robert Pear (December 26, 1987), © 1987.
North Carolina Medical Society for "A Checklist of Practice Marketing Ideas" by L. Beck and P. Salmon, *North Carolina Medical Journal* Vol. 46 p. 345, © 1985; and "Surviving in Today's Society" by D. Welton, *North Carolina Medical Journal* Vol. 28 p. 152, © 1967.
W. W. Norton & Co. for "The Changing Role of the Physician" by R. Ebert, in *Health Care and its Costs* , C. J. Schramm (editor), pp. 145-184, © 1987; and "The Loss of Innocence: Health Care Under Seige" by D. Cohodes, in Health Care and its Costs , C. J. Schramm (editor), pp. 64-104, © 1987.
Ohio State Medical Association for "Packaging Your Practice," *Ohio Medicine* Vol. 83 p. 769, © 1987; "Treating Your Practice - I," *Ohio Medicine* Vol. 83 p. 867, © 1987; "Treating Your Practice - II," *Ohio Medicine* Vol. 84 p. 49, © 1988; "Treating Your Practice - III," *Ohio Medicine* Vol. 84 p. 145, © 1988; and "Getting Professional Help," *Ohio Medicine* Vol. 84 p. 206, © 1988, all by the OSMA Department of Communications and Physician Marketing.
Daniel Okrent for "You and the Doctor: Striving for a Better Relationship, *The New York Times Magazine* (March 29, 1987), © 1987.
PR Publishing Co. for "Preparing for a TV Appearance," *PR Reporter* Vol. 17, © 1979; and "Basic Training Document: How You Look on TV May Be More Important Than What You Actually Say—Some Tips to Take With You to the Studio," *PR Reporter* Vol. 23, © 1985.
Prentice Hall for *Marketing for Health Care Organizations* by P. Kotler and R. Clarke, © 1987, p. 234.
Rhode Island Medical Society for "The Doctor as a Revolutionary: The Next Twenty-Five Years" by P. Mathieu, *Rhode Island Medical Journal* Vol. 58 p. 175, © 1975.
David E. Rogers for *Clinical Education and the Doctor of Tomorrow* , © 1988.
W. B. Saunders for "The Medical Interview and Related Skills" by M. Lipkin, *Office Practice of Medicine* , pp. 1287-1306, © 1987.

WGBH TV for "Can We Make a Better Doctor?" broadcast on *NOVA*, December 1988.
Williams and Wilkins for "The Doctor Image" by H. Bockus, *American Journal of Gastroenterology* Vol. 61 p. 356, © 1974.

Every effort has been made to obtain permission to use the material quoted in this book, and to trace all copyright holders. In the event of any question arising over the use of quoted material, however, the editor will be pleased to make the necessary correction in future printings.